Presence Perfect

Rita Bhimani is a public relations veteran with over forty years of dedicated experience. She is the founder of Ritam Communications, a PR consultancy, and also serves as a faculty member for a three-year degree course in Media Sciences.

In addition to her work in PR, Bhimani writes columns for various publications, has produced a documentary on Raja Rammohun Roy, and acts as a soft skills trainer. She's also known for hosting a range of industry events, literary readings, and celebrity interviews through her signature Red Sofa conversations.

Presence Perfect

Your Protein Boost for a Positive Image in 24 Doses

RITA BHIMANI

Published by
Rupa Publications India Pvt. Ltd 2025
7/16, Ansari Road, Daryaganj
New Delhi 110002

Sales centres:
Bengaluru Chennai Hyderabad
Jaipur Kathmandu Kolkata
Mumbai Prayagraj

Copyright © Rita Bhimani 2025

The views and opinions expressed in this book are the author's
own and the facts are as reported by her; these have been
verified to the extent possible, and the publishers are not
in any way liable for the same.

All rights reserved.
No part of this publication may be reproduced, transmitted,
or stored in a retrieval system, in any form or by any means,
electronic, mechanical, photocopying, recording or otherwise,
without the prior permission of the publisher.

P-ISBN: 978-93-7003-996-4
E-ISBN: 978-93-7003-250-7

First impression 2025

10 9 8 7 6 5 4 3 2 1

The moral right of the author has been asserted.

Printed in India

This book is sold subject to the condition that it shall not,
by way of trade or otherwise, be lent, resold, hired out, or otherwise
circulated, without the publisher's prior consent, in any form of
binding or cover other than that in which it is published.

*Dedicated to Kishore, my golden other,
the real writer amongst us.*

*'I Will Survive' has been his favourite song. I hope all my readers
will use survival strategies for their brand building.*

Contents

Introduction		*ix*
1	Amperage: The Singer, Not the Song	1
2	Anchorage: Maven Mentoring for Enhanced Net Worth	12
3	Advantage Age: The High Pitch of Life	21
4	Assemblage: Fulfilment of Life with Ikigai and Ichigo Ichie	30
5	Bandage: Setbacks as Springboards to Success	36
6	Courage: Techniques of a Techtonic Mind	43
7	Curettage: The Wellness of Medical Conviviality	51
8	Diplomage: Creating Coherence, Concord, Confluence	62
9	Engage: Riding the Radio Waves of Connectivity	71
10	Envisage: Clickbait in the Age of Influencers	79
11	Encourage: Mentoring Mindspace to Munificent Wealth-Share	88
12	Homage: Don't Walk Alone! Mentors Can Change Mindsets	95
13	Language: The Ramparts of Art	101
14	Laughage: Humour That Leavens Work Ethic	111

15	Linkage: Engaging through Music	120
16	Montage: Photogenic Travel Primping Empathetic Perception	127
17	Plumage: The Soft Feathers of Entrepreneurship	136
18	Rampage: Of Startups Serenaded by Angel Harps	144
19	Rivage: Transparent, Continuous, Cohesive Communication	152
20	Sportspage: Transformational, Not Just Inspirational	161
21	Verbiage: Letter Literacy—the Write Way	170
22	Voltage: Presentability over Mere Presence	178
23	Webpage: Of Social Media and Societal Connect	187
24	Weightage: Reimagining Brand Strategies Post Pandemic	195

Introduction

This book was conceived in cloistered Covid-tainted times, when difficulties were king-sized, solutions the reigning queen, and the knave of it all was our diffidence, and the misinformation that crowned it all. So, here we are with a book which sets out into this brave new world of ours, where 140 characters get you traction and a few seconds of tweeting, a big cache of money.

But there is still scope to talk, to write, to share from one's experience how image and presentability, and the ability to project one's ideas can gain you credibility, fame, power and self-esteem. And the impulse for staying the distance.

This is a 24-step protein boost for positive image creation. The book is all about the fact that while people may have learning and wisdom on their side, they may not always be able to give these talents the necessary fillip without an element of style. The 'perfect presence' matters. Erudition and wisdom are the Knowledge Quotient, or the KQ, one that forms the base, but it is the Preen Quotient, or the PQ, that is the glaze to draw the right gaze.

There is a lot to be said about sapience, which is the quality of being sagacious and discerning. We don't often play with this word and our usage is confined to the honorific we have given ourselves—homo sapiens, or loosely, 'wise human'. But the origin of sapience, we gather, is the Latin *sapientia*, meaning 'good taste', 'good sense', 'intelligence' or 'wisdom'.

Hence, sapience, the property of possessing wisdom, is one side of the coin of success in the business of life. The flip side—heads, actually—is the potency of style. Add to this self-esteem, selling power and staying the course, and you have the elements of perfect presence in positive play.

So, in today's post-Covid world, after everyone has learnt their lessons, coped with numerous lockdowns, assisted others, and braved and shaped their own destinies, with a little help from the vaccines that have given a modicum of assurance, this manual should serve to strengthen the resolve of stronger communication, better planning, and more focused ways to get ahead in a competitive environment.

Did you not count yourself amongst those millions who triumphantly posted pictures of taking the jab, as if to proclaim to the world that you had taken the first conquering step and then subsequently completed the process so you could be free to face the world, unbound?

The next logical step, thus, was to accept the vaccine factor as the big leap forward, with a new sense of the freeing up of mindsets. Moving from the individual perspective, the priorities then became work-related. Companies started encouraging employees to return to full-time work, and began to reverse the process of partial salaries. Businesses got their act together and venture capitalists came out of virtual confines to give a push to entrepreneurial dreams.

But while at the heart of it all has been the urge to rebuild, relearn and reconvene strategies, donning the hard hat of resolve, the approaches and methodology need the lacquer of practised presence, the style that can set you apart. That elusive patina of the perfection parquet.

This book is for those who are hard-pressed for time and need to have a quick dose of handheld, homegrown pragmatism.

Having been in the public relations profession, one is inclined to lean towards championing the idea of the 'preen' factor. It constitutes the swag of style that sits atop education, erudition and experience. That gains you an extra edge over competitors and co-workers. It is our belief that the preen and presentability factors can be as pivotal as wisdom and erudition.

Years ago, when my first book titled *The Corporate Peacock: New Plumes for Public Relations* was brought out by my current publishers, Rupa, the idea was to project the importance of the communication imperatives for companies onto a plumed world where their capabilities needed to be displayed. Somehow, nobody understood the word 'preen'.

Hence, I want to stress more on PQ, or the importance of the Preen Quotient in people's lives, with the same gravity as is required of a person's IQ and KQ. Intelligence and knowledge, yes, but applying that learning constitutes preen, or the ability to project and enhance this innate faculty.

Who preens? A peacock preens its feathers to show off its glorious colours. Yet, it is more than an act of narcissism. It is the peacock's way of sending out a mating signal, as the vibrant plumage is meant to attract and court the female. The more the patterned eyespots, the better the peacock's chance of getting more than one peahen to mate with.

In a wider context of preening reputation, a radiant and dynamic set of messages can get a more receptive target audience. An individual's ability to preen makes them stand apart and get noticed. And for a corporate entity, there can be no gainsaying the fact that preening should be a continuous process to ensure top-of-the-mind recall.

The new world of virtual and virile imperatives requires a fresh viridian ascendancy. It is one where the rules have to be tweaked by you, the individual who can make a difference, who can tackle the vicissitudes of the newly minted normalcy. I have chosen what I have christened as a 24-step protein boost, each step being an attempt to explore areas that seem obvious, but which many of us tend to be oblivious to, in the daily routine of formulating and formatting our circadian lifecycle.

Many of the pointers may appear to be basic and evident in daily life but they have been penned using the author's individual experiences and emprises to give you a digest of home truths and easy-to-ingest solutions. I have taken liberties with the term 'present perfect', for although one has been trained in the usage of participles and tenses in basic grammar studies, this phrase, I hope, will find a novel resonance.

In writing these homilies, I have occasionally used a word that is unusual, or created an aphorism that could seem highfalutin. The intention has not been to intimidate, but to get you to jump out of your skin regarding what you believe to be plainspeak. A turn of phrase, a twist of fate—let's see what upended 'communiquette' is all about.

Communication and the perfect visibility factor also embrace the various art forms—photography, painting, music and films, among others. Trawl through our various chapters to find what best works with serendipity in your life.

I have attempted to enmesh my personal experiences with expert-speak on many of the issues in the chapters. The interviews were done through email, Zoom, Google Meet and WhatsApp interactions—whichever platforms suited my respondents. Most of them are at the top of their professions and are extremely busy people, but none of them balked at giving me focused time. It is a measure of their professional commitment that gave me the confidence to move ahead and write. Nothing is done in isolation. The shared wisdom and the willing ampoules of knowledge have all been invaluable in giving *Presence Perfect* the heft it required.

The basis for having 'age' in the title of each chapter is *image*, which is what this book is all about.

The choice of 24 topics is to stress on the idea that the establishment of credible presence needs to be addressed 24/7. I hope the 24 ways and means can add to better productivity, more presentable projects, seminally successful projections and high-end impact. Stayin' alive, stayin' ahead. And also standing up and standing out are the messages.

When I advocate perfection, it is nothing but pre-planning, the pre-empting of possible crises, being impeccable in behaviour, exquisite in execution, precise in application, faultless in presenting your case, aiming for the acme of achievement, and a consummate and consistent ability to gain transcendence.

1

Amperage: The Singer, Not the Song

She has style, she has substance, she's the singer and the song
Her multi-structured communing is what has abided lifelong
The answer in the end
Is blowing in the wind
As the audiences continue at the hustings to throng

If ever there was someone who spelled connectivity in all forms, my vote, and that of scores of admirers, would go to Usha Uthup. Breaking the language, sound and audience barriers, keeping convention intact, yet challenging convention moulds, going that extra mile to sing, preach, bestow benefaction, and doing the 'P-to-P' on a daily basis. In my lexicon, that means People to People, Preen to Perfection, and Planning till Posterity.

So, here will be another 'P'—poetically writing this chapter in eight sonnets, each set signifying the focal points of her career. The singer who, at all times, believes in the power of connecting, creating, conversing, communing and contemporizing.

In this chapter, quite different in approach from the rest of the chapters that follow, we attempt to bring in a poetic twist in describing the communicability of a person who has become an institution in the world of music for over half a century. Wherever she goes, she is met with adulation and admiration, and there are legions of people who will have their favourite Usha tale to share. A well-known journalist and author, Vikas Kumar Jha even spent several years on penning a warm biography on her, with the joyous title *Ullas Ki Naav*, released by top celebs in 2020. It took me three months to go through the fat tome, and have conversations with Jha, apart from sessions with Usha herself, but at the end, there were hundreds of stories that were unearthed, which I, as someone who has known her for 50 years, found new, revealing and inspirational. There's never a cause she has not touched, never a skill which she has not perfected, never a request she has turned down, and she is ever the one to connect from the heart, sing from the soul.

What about a biopic on you, I asked. Would you play you? 'Yes, unabashedly, yes' was her guileless response. But the strong family person she is, her next answer hit the right notes too. The young Usha would be played by daughter Anjali (a seasoned presenter) of course, and the earliest Usha could be granddaughter Aisha.

While much of the facts about her life are in the public domain, I decided to contain some special facets into an octagonal tribute, which hopefully will have its own lyrical tilt. There's poetic licence in the songs I have placed in the eight different sonnets as far as chronological acuity is concerned.

Why eight? It is her lucky number, signifying her birth date. It is also a number that symbolizes harmony and balance and abundance and power. In China, it spells prosperity. Why—the Beijing Olympics began on 8 August 2008 at eight seconds and eight minutes past 8 p.m.! So eight it will be.

May there be, as the Beatles said, 'Eight Days a Week' to calibrate this singing sensation, on whom has been conferred the Padma Bhushan.

Facet One: Passioning Music

She believes in music, and she believes in love,
It's deep down inside her, and her manna from above.
When first she belted 'Fever', the year was sixty-nine,
'Jambalaya' was so rapturous, made the Madras folks supine!
She was just twenty-one, and at Silver Sands she crooned,
She sang a Tamil song and oh! How the audience swooned.

So lesson one, she learnt from then which she in life did heed,
That music has no barriers, nor any caste, colour or creed.
Her persona was the girl next door, but she took 'Savera' by storm,
She sang 'Haal Kaisa Hai Janaab Kaa'—as South turned northwards norm.
She struck the right connecting chords and made a people music niche,
So versatile, an Indophile, who succeeded in multi-language breach.
She never learnt the formal way, but radio music gave her spark,
To pursue jazz, rock, pop and ethnic and on life's work to embark.

Facet Two: Prime Time

So many crooners came and went, but Usha stood above the rest,
As Park Street swung to rock and pop from a voice enriched with zest.
A maiden on the maidan with her guitar she did with passion strum,
'Auld Acquaintance' in Bangla, which got the crowds in upward hum.

Then on to Trincas where she held all with her rock and pop,
And gave her heart to Jani in a brand new name to prop.
We jammed the place with coffees shared to hear music divine,
Her twinkling eyes and richset voice dipped us in sweet salt brine.

Those were the Trincas days which drew great celeb folks,
The filmdom stars, and politicos too, as she attracted gals and blokes.
And belted out 'Those Were The Days' and 'Matilda' took her beat,
And they 'Listened to the Pouring Rain', and wore their virtual dancing feet.

So full fifty years hence she came right back, and was received with acclaim,
The unstoppable Usha was ever new, of 'Skyfall' in a saree fame.

Facet Three: Performance, Performance, Performance

She was the playback prima, as large films got their prepped distaff,
From *Shalimar* and *Disco Dancer* to the hit movie *7 Khoon Maaf*.
'Hare Rama Hare Krishna' was her first big break,
From then on, it was hers to command and filmy orders to slake.

Her 'One Two Cha Cha Cha' still gives us beat, as does 'Rambha Ho',
But it's her heartful 'Darrrling' that gave the movie so much glow.
It is still one of her tribute numbers as the lady she still sings the blues,
While 'Auva Auva, Hari Om Hari', 'Uri Uri Baba' set our senses loose.

Performance also includes her acting, in *7 Khoon Maaf* she had character role,
In all the others she played herself, but with a commitment that none could troll.
From jingles to children's tales, and stage appearances the world over,
It's the pulse of the people she always felt which kept her on connective clover.

In seventeen Indian languages and many foreign ones she's been a sensation,
'Malaika' in Swahili made the Kenyan President give her the keys to the nation.

Facet Four: Priming Vibrations, Premiering Awards, Padma Bhushan

For the manifaceted Usha, she went beyond the staging of shows,
To setting up the very heart of a place where music truly grows.
And so Studio Vibrations was born, though earlier big ads were done from home,
But to vibrations all great musicians flocked for their multi-tracked work to hone.

Salil Choudhury, Asha Bhosle, Ravi Shankar were all there,
It was a hub and a heartland which gave musicians tech and care.
There's commerce, sure, but something else as young musicians find hope,
To come and grow their talents here and increase their success scope.

Much later was another deed which shows Usha's vision in macro light,
As she initiated Technicians awards, to recognize the people who had the right.
To have their work behind the scenes applauded in public gaze,
The Stagecraft awards- another big leap by her, brought in encouragement blaze.

Awards for her came thick and fast, but the one crowning glory was the one,
Which came conferred as Padma Bhushan to someone who had stunned the sun.

Facet Five: Papal Blessings

These other facets are of Usha, who embodies the secular tenet to a T,
But first, see how she was received by the Pope himself at Vatican See.
Teresa had been part of her life for four decades and more,
So the sainthood tribute that she gave was the song 'Poorest of the Poor'.

Tim Sebastian from BBC quickly got Usha for minutes three,
And in that time, Usha said, she learnt the art of brevity.
She came back armed with rosaries, all blessed by the Pope,
It was her way of sharing moments and giving us all special hope.

She is truly multi-faithed, as we've seen over the decades long,
Her goddess Saraswati shines bright in her studio, with veena, mike and song.
At Christmas, she bakes a hundred cakes and distributes to one and all,
And Onam sees her expertise in churning out the harvest thrall.
The gods and goddesses reside in harmony in her melodic home,
Epitomizing what secular really means, in the lexicon of her tenets dome.

Facet Six: Paparazzi Pet

The paparazzi we mention here is the people who follow her where she goes,
At restaurants, or at public spots, in hotels, hospitals, and in movies shows.
On our annual puja parikramas, the strangest sights we got to see,
When instead of focus on the goddess, the public found in her a Devi.

She wears this fame quite lightly, though, and with the public she can spar,
She's as much a people's person as on world platforms she is the star.
Her kanjeevaram classics, her bejewelled look, her bindi and that smile,
Complete with kanjeevaram sneakers give her both glamour and guile.

She's presented her cobblers on stage, to the President of India too,
There's no one who comes into her ken who does not get their due.
She's generous to a fault, and her philanthropy is unbounded,
She plans the perfect picnics, parties with joyous abandon unfounded.

Nothing mundane about these, because it shows her grounded ways,
Of mucking in, and melding with friends and keeping them ever in gaze.

Facet Seven: Primping Friendships

When chips were down in Covid crunch, she proved a superstar,
As she looked well beyond her own fame to give our hopes a spar.
Throughout the lockdown never did she let the spirits pall,
Of our gang of girls, diverse, but close, for whom she gave creative thrall.

She started with the Puja beat, in our own homes she made us dance,
Her demo videos prepped us up and endgame saw all in dervish trance.
More performances did she bring to fore, as she made us do much more,
From hula dance to the latest prance as 'Jerusalema' put us on show.

And then, to allay people's fears of Covid's far-reaching pace,
A song sung in our many voices saw us also ace.
The inspiring 'Hum Ko Mann Ki Shakti Dena' made us double braves,
A professional offering that got massive following on the social media waves.
Divas we all ended up, feeling preened and primped with fame,
As Uthopian Usha stood back with pride and let the rest claim flame!

Facet Eight: Pacesetter among Professionals

The Covid times and lockdown limits made Usha introspect to core,
To nix sad state and convert it to strengths with which to explore.
How to connect by stayin' alive, alert and doing shows galore,
At home full set-up she created, a studio space right at the fore.

In full regalia she would always appear, with stars sparkling in the set,
And that is how she taught stagecraft, through blank screens doing connect.
The shows she did were toppers all, which covered US cities coast to coast,
It was hard work, but viewers adored it all, and she stayed uppermost.

She did more shows, recordings during lockdown than in the last ten years,
She believes communication is her business and music allays all fears.
Connectivity is her true strength, and we will never see her charisma pall,
The biography on her *Ullas Ki Naav* shows her in glorious thrall.

She is the singer beyond the song, the perfectionist, melody queen,
The thinker, performer, doer, who can never lose her sheen.

This chapter brings out the polygonal facets of communication, which have been presented in the rest of the book through a focus on people and institutions ranging from art to IT, from education to social media, from branding to bespoke travel. Check into whatever catches your fancy.

2

Anchorage: Maven Mentoring for Enhanced Net Worth

Why a Pride of Lions but a Prejudice with female
Why the haughty male gaze, when she's top of the dale
She's the ten-handed one
Who can go stun the sun
But is always in scrutiny if she were ever to fail

In the prescriptive chapters that have been ideated, the objective is to make the panaceas universal. Meaning, no gender bias. But how can I, as a woman author, not be able to give vent to some areas of concern and of opportunity for women—in this case, networking. While everyone needs to network, I am specially seized of the fact that the difference lies in perception.

In fact, in writing this woman-centric chapter, I would encourage the reader to consider the word 'maven', which stands for someone who is an acknowledged expert in a given field, and more importantly, who shares their knowledge with others. The feminine twist to this is that maven is often used to mean a female expert!

So, we move to some deep-seated prejudiced viewpoints. When a woman talks of networking, she is considered to be a social butterfly. And there's a term used with such insouciance in this context that I wonder why it is not erased from our vocabulary: the socialite! You step a little out of your crease to make an individual statement and there you are, caught in the glare of arc lamps and a posse of paparazzi. The bimbette without a brief. Or the barely clad bitch. It appears to have become a moniker for a person from the upper social echelons (whatever that means!) who revolves in high-end circles attending parties, events, can entertain with aplomb, and speak her mind at charity events. She has a discrete (and here I point you to a word which means 'separate') calling and in her time, plays many parts; bless Shakespeare.

No, the networking that we are talking about is for women in professions who need to get out and mingle—proffer business cards, drink, talk, ideate and build connections—in the process exchanging information, often discussing politics or the state of the economy or areas of mutual cultural interest. When the guys are seen to be in these furtherment conversations, they are looked at as dynamic and serious, even if they happened to be discussing the next day's racing fixtures or gossiping about the 'beautiful' new corporate entrant, whereas a woman in these conversational connects is perceived to be on a soft-power pitch.

Then, here's the crunch. Doesn't the same networking help the working woman get difficult things done? Is the aggressive stance of a woman executive taken to be of a brazen hussy? Not anymore. And who could be a better person to focus on this than Mumbai-based businesswoman and author Apurva Purohit, who, with more than 30 years of corporate experience, showed how she could form great partnerships with private equity firms and promoters to build and scale up a diverse set of business. Right up to supervising turnarounds in mature and declining organizations. Her LinkedIn profile also states: 'She has worked across a variety of media businesses from radio to print to digital, and was responsible for building and scaling up *Radio City*, setting up Lodestar, one of the largest media buying agencies in the country, and envisioning *The Times of India*'s entry strategy into television. She has also worked on famed turnarounds like *Zee TV* and *Mid-Day*.' She recently co-founded Aazol Ventures Pvt Ltd—a consumer products company which sells traditional food items made by self-help groups and micro entrepreneurs—with her son, Siddharth Purohit.

And more importantly, the person who has, from huge personal experience, given large amounts of hope and advice, through her national bestselling books: *Lady, You're not a Man—the Adventures of a Woman at Work* and *Lady, You're the Boss*.

For someone who has been ranked as one of the most powerful women in business over many successive years, her words need to be inhaled deeply, smoked if you must, and internalized. She's that maven we talked about in the beginning of this chapter. The word, incidentally, comes from the Yiddish word 'mevyn', which means 'one who understands'. However, it has to go beyond mere understanding, and a maven is really an expert who has garnered knowledge over time and to whom people turn for their expertise.

She starts out by insisting on not demeaning the word 'networking' and wanting women to look at not deprioritizing this by saying that they are pressed for time. They don't want to be caught socializing, you see. Purohit wants a message to go out to women: 'Networking is, actually, being able to connect with people from whom you can learn and to whom you can give. Connections help both sides grow. You have to network in industry forums. You should also get out of your own department and mingle in other departments to get a better idea of other disciplines. If you are a senior person, you need to network with your juniors. It is all about building connections.'

There is plenty of learning to be had from this sort of interaction and a teaching element too. Relationships can then become mutually beneficial. More so, for women who should live life on their own terms.

There is an incident that Purohit recounts about how she wanted to bring in a humanizing factor into a mundane meeting. Imagine the surprise and horror of the largely all-male executives—who had prepared their plans for the beginning of the week offering—to be faced with a pretty cake with icing and edible pink roses. While having their portions, they also had to share how their weekend went in terms of non-work. It was her way of bringing out their real persona. Although this was largely a male-dominated morning, it also served to get women to air their authentic selves. The freewheeling chat also made for defusing tensions and created a sense of trust. This is where the making of winning teams had a beginning.

'Be who you are. Do not play to the protective nature of men colleagues, or try to be a man yourself in an effort to be part of the club. And in the long run, with women being perfectionists, as a result of multi-tasking, there is also the sincerity and commitment that comes to the fore.'

She believes that they must become the torchbearers of self-worth and the upending of personal identity. Purohit is clear about the 'perform or perish' syndrome, as women have had to fight harder to be where they are and therefore must take their responsibilities more seriously. Vocal and visible are the key elements if you have to belong to the centre of the table. When we try to take a peek into Apurva Purohit's own approaches to her successful career, she talks with conviction using just three points to illustrate her methodology.

'I work very hard to be authentic. I am not shy about hiding my good and bad points and hence, there is no web of deceit that is woven. When you are authentic and not posturing or pretending to be what you are not, it removes any stress on yourself. You have to project self-confidence, which comes out of self-esteem. The second is that I add value to people's lives. You could say I am more of a coach and a trainer and less of a boss in the traditional sense. That is how engaged teams are built. And finally, I have a sense of clarity and am able to simplify chaos. I approach all our business with a uniform, strategic consistency.'

For someone with 30 per cent women in her workforce, which is quite the acceptable norm today, Purohit's message is that you do not need to have large titles to be strong influencers. You need empathy and authenticity and of course, the end-game of the presentability push to make a mark. Management by example is the Purohit philosophy which other women who are leading the pack in numerous enterprises are doing with élan.

So, here I would like to serve up some of the wisdom distilled from Apurva Purohit's *Lady, You're the Boss*, to reiterate five key points:

1. Push the boundaries of your potential.
2. Step out of the perception bias.
3. Co-opt men into the diversity conversation.
4. Live unabashedly, loudly, walking with pride.
5. Multitask for yourself, to build your own net worth.

There is also a leadership style which propels the female workforce, whether it be senior executives or their junior counterparts, to understand the nuances of strictures, and a parenting attitude. Management by listening, in the case of Purohit's approach, is not just an academic concept, but is practised with focused intent to get into the psyche of executives. The use of tough-love techniques has also been a factor for instilling a can-do attitude, where killing with kindness is replaced with unsentimental strictness to enable people to buck up and find their own solutions, sans the pampering. The individualistic approach and the scaling up have resulted in a re-energized workforce.

Something that may still lurk within us when this book emerges in physical form is the Covid-19 virus and its fallout. When it was surging, a group of women lawyers met through a networking community on LinkedIn, and the result was an anthology where these hotshot legal eagles (I wonder why we always append 'hotshot' to lawyers? Must start some other charged-up terminology for other professions) focused on many aspects of work experience. The title of the book says it pithily: *#Networked: How 20 Women Lawyers Overcame the Confines of Covid Social Distancing to Create Connections, Cultivate Community, & Build Businesses in the Midst of a Global Pandemic.*

They covered a wide range of topics and this book is meant to serve as an inspiration to women professionals. The pandemic was seen as a boost to opportunity and augmentation. To quote from the 'Introduction' to the book by Shari E. Belitz, 'the pandemic wasn't a time of destruction at all. No, it was the birth of a whole new me, or rather a whole new *we*.' The electronic medium that bonded them, LinkedIn, went 'across state lines, social circles, religions, generational groups, socioeconomic status and political views.' They found commonalities and expanded their networks to include more diverse perspectives. The unique thing they did was going for 'net-weaving' in preference to networking. In her piece, Jamie Szal, an attorney who specializes in taxation, expands on what her friend from the Women's Leadership Council offered by way of explanation. 'Net-weaving is the idea that women, in many ways, take pride in and intentionally seek out opportunities to be a point of connection for other women, weaving threads in a larger tapestry of women supporting women in their professional goals.'

Talking about women supporting advancement of women addressing the issue of unequal pay, we have economic historian and Harvard University professor Claudia Goldin who won the Noble Prize in Economic Sciences in 2023. The prize recognizes her pioneering research on our understanding of labour market outcomes for women. Basically, that women are hopelessly under-represented in the world of work, and while their numbers are growing, wages are much lower than those of men. Goldin is the first woman to get the prize solo. Her research is heartening for us, pointing to two factors that are essential to bringing more women into the workforce—higher education investments and raising the age of marriage.

Author's afterthoughts: In the process of talking from my high writer-horse, I must admit to my own failed networking, or net-weaving nadirs. It's another country, another world—that of academia. It is the university-town of Athens, Georgia, and I am in the company of 40 students from far-flung countries, all of us there on a student scholarship. I am the only Indian girl and the others are from Norway, Sweden, Iceland, Denmark, Germany, Austria, Taiwan, Japan, Iran—too many to remember now. Yes, there lies the rub. We form close friendships, some of us even banding together to tour most of the US, Mexico and Canada by car, pitching tents. They are of diverse hues—a German who is an art history major, an Austrian from nobility, a European who claims to have ballet-danced with [Rudolf] Nureyev, my Japanese roommate who fiercely overcame language problems to write her thesis, etc. But what if these relationships had been capitalized on and the connections maintained over distances. The world would have been my oyster!

Neither did I keep up with the Jamshedpur biggies, nor later, in my working life, with the professional leaders of industry, post my taking the icy leap forward in my own consultancy after a comforting cocoon of corporate complacence with a multinational. The only satisfaction—that work came to me without marketing myself and the execution of nearly three decades of creative work done with a measure of consistency, I hope, and without unseemly dreams of attaining popularity or fame.

The 'what-if' remorse comes to the fore now and then, when post Covid, many people are no more—those I would have liked to pick up the threads with, in the context of this book. There are, of course, small linkages which show that old girls' networks can be revived by just pressing the enter key. After nearly two decades, I sent a blind email to Kaarina Alanko in Helsinki, a respected counterpart in the International Public Relations circuit and one of the few International Public Relations Association (IPRA) woman presidents. I needed to find out about the large proportion of women in the new Finnish cabinet headed by a woman prime minister. In the process of our emailed conversations, it emerged that women leaders have their cabinet meetings in the saunas that are a central part of the Finnish culture. With this, a whole new article was created and plenty of memories revived of a professional PR trip that fuelled the idea for setting up a consultancy firm for me.

The reason for this back story is to emphasize just one point, and that is, in the context of this chapter, **to focus on net worth and never take networking for granted. Let linkages happen with more solidity than through mere Instagrammed posts.** And in that process, let's close the inequity gap.

3

Advantage Age: The High Pitch of Life

When you've performed on every premiere stage
And your life's work has glorious plumage
Your words take on heft
As you weave warp and weft
Into the fabric of inspiration for gen-next to engage

One of the singular joys of my life has been to be able to climb the age ladder and get to the near-top rung, to connect with the grand-age people of eminence. Ninety and above, nimble and nifty, in the way they continue to keep up their passions, their demanding work routines, and their discipline in leading a life that is beyond evanescence—exemplary in all aspects and inspirational to the hilt.

When I first launched into a series called the *Red Sofa Conversations*, it was an idea that came from Harshvardhan and Madhu Neotia—the innovative thrust from one of them and the creative spark from the other to carry it forward. The venue was their very own The Conclave, the first-ever exclusive business club in Kolkata, which became an epicurean venue too. The dubbing of the term 'Red Sofa' was by Naveen Kishore, publisher extraordinaire. We, literally, had a red sofa where I was to sit to have one-on-one interactions with celebrities from variegated walks of life. A warm, intimate, communicative platform with a handpicked audience for good measure.

Having steered through twenty such celebs that included authors, film directors and actors, political personages, sportspeople, singers, fashion designers, artists and journalists, there came a stage when I felt it was time to get to another level and do a sub-set titled 'Life Peaks at Ninety'.

The first one to come to the Red Sofa was danseuse Amala Shankar. At 95, there she was, elegantly turned out in her signature burnished gold garad silk, beatifically beaming at the audience, and practically ready to get up and demonstrate a few dance steps. She had also given birth to a brand new talent—drawing and painting. A large body of her work was displayed and up for sale too at the Academy of Fine Arts. Never did she put a *step* wrong while sharing anecdotes as she plucked them out of her memory bank—from her early days of meeting husband Uday Shankar and keeping his gharana alive through their daughter Mamata and daughter-in-law Tanusree, to playing the role of King Janaka in the dance drama *Sita Swayamvar* when she was 92 and walking the red carpet at 94 at the Cannes Film Festival where the iconic film featuring her and Uday Shankar, *Kalpana* (1948), was screened. She lived to be 100.

We go back to sharing the wisdom of the ninety-pluses, as their creative construct never seems to ebb.

I have imbibed several lessons in the course of the writing of this book and conducting interviews. The more accomplished an individual is, the more graciously and ungrudgingly they share their time.

Balkrishna Doshi, who passed last January, was an architect

visionaire. Every time one met him, one felt deeply fulfilled. I have followed his work and seen it in its physical reality or realty, if you will, over the decades. He has always had time to talk, to share higher thoughts, to laugh, to be down to the very earth, which he feels gives him resurgence.

His architecture, his vision, his approach to living spaces and to the aesthetics of life, his deep scholarship, and his wide reach with over 100 projects that defy the spatial conventions, how else would the world have recognized such a man but by conferring on him the prestigious Pritzker Architecture Prize in 2018. It is equivalent to receiving a Nobel in Architecture and he is the only Indian to have been given this award. The jury talked about 'his commitment and his dedication to his country and the communities he has served, his influence as a teacher, and the outstanding example he has set for professionals and students around the world throughout his long career.' Most of all, they referred to him as someone 'demonstrating substantial contributions to humanity, for over 60 years.'

This is at the heart of his creations—his projects going 'beyond the functional to connect with the human spirit through poetic and philosophical underpinnings.' Yes, he was influenced by internationally renowned architects like Le Corbusier and Louis Kahn (and loved the quirkiness, beauty and joy of [Spanish architect Antoni] Gaudi's architecture, he had once told me), but his was an ethical and personal approach to architecture, and he was the person who was 'instrumental in shaping the discourse of architecture throughout India and internationally.'

When I asked him to share the new vocabulary he had created by harmonizing history and culture, local traditions and the changing Indian scenario, this master of philosophical simplification said: 'Every day trees change, I take my lessons from nature, from the celebrations, fluctuations and opportunities.'

As a mentor, when he met students, he raised his hand and then stretched it forward. 'I do not stand erect but I bend slightly. So I remove the notion of separation. I ask them about their work and their discovery. How do you bring association, connection, relationship and the kind of opening for them to talk unless you come down to their level? I come off the stage and speak to people.'

Talking of 'projects going beyond the functional to connect with the human spirit,' he said that the answer is not only dialogue but getting into the skin of others. 'Don't stand apart. You must feel you belong to them through gestures of behaviour and relationships.'

'What is the whole idea of belonging and togetherness? If I create an object, I try to create the sense of belonging and memories. Because architecture is a living thing. It does not function in isolation. My architecture shakes hands. How can a building embrace the surrounding? This is when the dialogue starts. There has to be a beauty and necessity of open spaces. Like relationships. Of animating things. Why should a building be separate from you?'

'If you do not have the multidimensional vision or the temperament of doing what you are best at, can you achieve anything?'

This is exactly what we are advocating as communicators.

When we asked him about sharing his wisdom and wealth, he spoke of togetherness being wealth in the same manner as rejoicement is. 'Together is the joy of life.' At the heart of it all is working with commitment, creativity and continuity. He signed off by saying, 'Celebrate what you do. Celebrate what you think and share it. Live naturally and be part of the universe. You are never born poor. You have been given eyes and ears and a body. You are born with abundance.'

We have received abundant joy of living benediction from this Aaronic architect, dapper in appearance, diehard in demeanour, and soft-centred in his outreach, activating life's sensibilities through a shared greatness.

Another of the ninety-plus nifty nabobs featured on *Red Sofa Conversations* comes from a completely different segment. Again, an individual whom I have observed over the years where his wise counsel never flags.

A.C. Chakrabortti is a doyen in the chartered accountancy firmament. When he conducts his business, not just of his own firm but as the director of innumerable reputed companies, his voice is heard, his opinions taken and implemented to their benefit, and his presence feared, revered and commandeered.

Having been on the board of one of the companies where he has frequently taken the chair, I had a chance to observe, up close and personal, the methodology of his approach, the trust he generated, and the wisdom that made the company sit up and take note of course correction. He has suffered my ignorance on financial matters, but has been immensely encouraging of my writing, even going to the trouble of giving his comments on Amazon for my last PR book (*PR 2020: The Trending Practice of Public Relations*), which many close friends failed to do, out of sheer ennui.

ACC (as we will refer to him throughout this chapter, for Chakrabortti seems impertinent, journalistically correct though it may be) has no such succumbing to the listless. He is ever at the green light, in attitude, appearance and work ethic.

That's the goal of this book—to keep ahead, stay the distance, and add optimistic grains of sugar and salt to personal goals, to corporate intent.

He does not just talk from his commanding heights, but loves to go back to his time in S.R. Batliboi & Co. when he became a partner in the firm because he always believed in the excellent mentors there who moulded him into the hugely successful professional that he is today. Being the leader of the team which negotiated with Ernst & Young, ACC found that experience to be highly rewarding and satisfying. But when he had to comment on leadership, he always gave the stage to partners, saying that everyone contributed to growth in diverse ways.

There are gems from our conversation vis-à-vis the book where he actively participated in answering every question of mine. He rued the fact that a lot of companies today lack vision and are unable to read the future and project it. You need talented people in the company for image building, for benefits to accrue in the long run, and this was aimed particularly at family-run corporations. The outlook of the management must be visionary in order to allow meritorious people to come, who must then progress with the company. For someone so senior, his harping on the need for keeping up with technology is heartening.

'Technology will change the way business is being transacted today. And the methodology of using it must go hand in hand. The world is changing very fast and long-stayers in companies are at a premium.'

He feels it is for the HR heads to play a vital role in succession analysis, which is important for sustaining the future.

'A lot of young people leave companies for better benefits in other places, but if remuneration systems are improved, of course with targets in place and even stock options, there could be less attrition rates.

'A good company is one where the employees feel proud of their company. Good communication must be an integrated part of the company's operation. There must be continued effort to motivate, something that is management's obligation to them.

'Employees do understand when a company is not doing well, but management must try to revive the company so that employees can be part of the joint endeavour to ensure [the] revival of [the] company. Corporates must be prepared to change their business culture. I can recount a case when the chairman of a company was the promoter and he insisted on paying salaries to all employees throughout the difficult period when others were putting in cutbacks. Finance pleaded for a cut in salaries but the chairman said they must pay the full amount. Holding back salaries does not impact the bottom-line in any significant way.'

We lauded ACC for reaching a wonderful age at which he could be sitting back and enjoying his leisure time but no, he continues to be extremely active, always prepared to the letter for board meetings through doing extensive preparation to make the meetings more actionable. 'I want to give a message to the younger lot that they should not hang up their boots at 40, but continue to grow, share, look for new pastures.'

Finally, ACC believes in hard work, perseverance and persistence, with luck playing a small part in all this.

This is a chapter without end! We could not stop at the nineties milestone. For on the scene appeared a most comely, gracious individual—Aditi Mukerjea, all of 102!

In a rare face-to-face interview that I took for *The Telegraph*, Mukerjea shared stories that had the stamp of conviction, topped up with humour and replete with the historic narrative of someone who had witnessed a nation undergoing change. She imbibed the heritage of her grandfather, Deshbandhu Chittaranjan Das, ingested the tradition and values of the Swaraj movement, and inspired by grandmother Basanti Devi, and subsequently her mother Sujata Devi, nurtured and transformed an orphanage.

In recounting the growth and development of the Sujata Devi Vidyamandir, Mukerjea shared with us a fascinating part of history when Mahatma Gandhi came into the picture.

It was the grim times of the infamous Noakhali riots. Sujata Devi had started an orphanage at a time she had sadly lost one of her own children, and Gandhiji sent six Hindu girls for rehabilitation. That was the beginning of the Bangiya Pallee Sangathan Samity. The orphanage finally morphed into a meaningful school, which got recognition in 1953 and thence became a college.

Mukerjea packs a pretty punch when she narrates all this, saving the juiciest bits that form a part of the growth of Sujata Devi Sadan. The year was 1973 and *Bobby* was premiering. Raj Kapoor—a family friend—happened to be on the scene. It collected a whopping ₹2 lakh, all of which was given to the school, one which still continues to serve the community.

Riveting, too, are the tales of Mukerjea's grandmother, Basanti Devi, the grande dame wife of Deshbandhu Chittaranjan Das, on whom was conferred the Padma Vibhushan—the second-highest civilian honour. Her grandmother lived up to the age of 95, and encouraged husband C.R. Das to continue his legal practice which was highly lucrative. But he gave it up to join the Swaraj movement, and so did her grandmother—Thakuma—who, along with her sister, a lifelong widow, was jailed. It was the English governor who came and got them out.

Basanti Devi believed neither in having statues of her husband nor in changing names of roads. So Nafar Kundu Road, where Mukerjea and her family live, still continues to have that name. Nafar Kundu was a sewage worker, who heroically risked his own life when he went into a manhole to save two other sewage workers trapped inside. A Hindu sacrificing his life for Muslims!

Mukerjea's deep political commitments saw her casting her vote uninterrupted from 1952.

Her mind so clear, credit given to others, and her activity of continuing to knit for her great grandchildren—maybe that's what keeps her glowing with an amazing grace, and luminous is the aura that she gives out. A fulfilling journey where age is just a statistic and not static at that. She continues in alert mode, mellow, empathetic, in sync with friends and family, content to have imbibed the highs and lows of a whole century.

So, fear not the advent of age—it merely enhances and sharpens the accumulated experience of life.

4

Assemblage: Fulfilment of Life with Ikigai and Ichigo Ichie

Enjoy this moment
For it will not come again
If you value life

While all our other chapters start with a limerick, here is a deviation since it is about 'ikigai'. Hence, the haiku as our header. With its strict seventeen syllables in three lines of five, seven and five, it has an emotive discipline. Significant, as we will talk about a particular philosophy of life that our fast-paced world can grasp like a falling star in one's palm and imbibe its magical and deep power of the now and here.

There are so many ways that we can get to clutch the perfection path. And edge nearer to the search for a meaningful life that has a defined purpose and leads a person to fulfilment. Nothing utopian about it. In fact, one of the gentlest and yet highly purposeful concepts that we have come across is the Japanese 'ikigai'. It is not exactly what we, in India, would call yogic, but it is close to yoga when you look at ikigai as a way of life, as something that denotes a long and happy journey through life.

The quiet elegance, the understated style, the effortless grouting in tradition all meshed in with an innate joyous presentiment—could this be a microcosm of 'ikigai' as a way of life?

As I once sat down to the partaking of a multi-course lunch, a splendid spread of everything from Norwegian salmon teriyaki and delicate tempura, to varied sushi and sashimi, with former Japanese Consul General in Kolkata, Yutaka Nakamura, many of the questions about what ikigai really means came across in genteel morsels of revelation. There was relentless rain outside that afternoon, reminding one of the beginning of *The Book of Ichigo Ichie: The Art of Making the Most of Every Moment, the Japanese Way*, where the authors are sipping a bright green infusion in a teahouse with the rain pounding the cobblestones. But where we were dining, with the quiet elegance of Japanese hospitality, the driving rain did not intrude into calm conversation and chopsticked culinary comfort.

While us outsiders, 'the gaijin' in Japanese, are all revved up about the concept of ikigai, through an earlier book *Ikigai: The Japanese Secret to a Long and Happy Life* by Héctor García and Francesc Miralles, what does it signify to someone who is a native Japanese, and maybe someone to whom it could just signal a way of life?

I had asked a rather simplistic query of Yutaka Nakamura, about when he was exposed to ikigai and how important it was in his line of profession as a diplomat. His answer to this was a neatly tailored approach: 'When I was little, I was wondering what I was born for. I became interested in what was happening around me and the situation in the world, and began to think deeply about peace. And later, I became aware of my job as a diplomat. Something that is tough, both mentally and physically, and I need to maintain strong motivation, so I think it is important to find an ikigai in the job.'

He went on to elaborate: 'I have never been aware of the philosophy of ikigai. I think that the concept of ikigai is, unconsciously, a part of life for Japanese people. So, as a diplomat, I can keep away from the distractions of constantly evolving external factors if I keep the axis of protecting the interests of the people and contributing to peace.'

We got the whole feel of ikigai, not so much by what was said, but what was unspoken, when we learnt that practising ikigai does mean how one can define a purpose, a personal mission and vision, and then let it translate into one's full potential. Someone told us, 'The aim is to define what you can best contribute to the world, what you're good at, and what you enjoy doing. Those who are actively working to discover their ikigai have shown [to display a] higher self-esteem and a feeling [that] their presence in the world is justified.'

This meeting with the Japanese Consul General was something that I would term as my 'ichigo ichie' moment, that is, once-in-a-lifetime meeting to cherish. The Japanese believe that what we are experiencing right now will never happen again; hence it is important to value each moment like a beautiful treasure. The Japanese also believe in being meticulous in their hospitality, which the guest must be sensitive enough to grasp and to accept in that spirit. We learnt that one should enjoy every encounter to the fullest.

And so one moves on to 'ichigo ichie', in the context of the corporate world. Surprisingly, one of the CEOs in a large FMCG firm had not only read the book, but also talked about how they had sessions through the HR department about the happiness quotient for employees. Each employee needs to be in a role with daily tasks that are aligned with their own personal and professional purpose, which results in greater life

Assemblage: Fulfilment of Life with Ikigai and Ichigo Ichie

fulfilment. We have to see what the word stands for. 'Ikiru' means life, and 'kai', loosely translated, is the realization one hopes for. So, many people describe 'ikigai' as 'a reason to get up in the morning'. Therefore, when individual ikigais are aligned with workplace goals, an employee is following the process of creating a fulfilling organization.

A lot of others have started 'living' some of the truths of *Ichigo Ichie*, another book written by the authors of *Ikigai*. They talk about learning to make every moment a 'once-in-a-lifetime experience'.

In their book *Ichigo Ichie*, the authors talk about the idea of observing and cherishing each moment and the practice of harnessing that attention to achieve harmony with others and love life. They say, 'The teachings of Zen, the Japanese version of Buddhism, give us many opportunities to incorporate "Ichigo Ichie" into our daily lives.'

And in the process they give eight guidelines 'for honing the power of observation'. Some of these are: to embrace the moment; savour this moment as being the best moment of your life; avoid distractions—do one thing at a time ('a hunter who takes aim at two preys at once will kill none'); free yourself from everything that isn't essential; assume that you are unique in the world; understanding that it's perfect to be imperfect; realizing that feeling sorry for someone doesn't mean feeling pity but rather a profound empathy; and letting go of your expectations. Ichigo Ichie is experienced with the uncluttered mind taught by Zen.

We are further given an insight into the ten principles that sum up this Japanese philosophy. We are told that life is a question of now or never as each opportunity presents itself only once. Of course, you are urged to live as if this were going to happen just once in your life. Dwelling in the present is encouraged, as is doing something you have never done before, and of course, in the process you cannot forget to practise meditation and add mindfulness to your five senses; be aware of coincidences; make every day a celebration; reinventing yourself is prime and keeping up the practice, so that the more abundant the results will be.

For many of us in the corporate world, our early diet used to be based on the precepts of 'kaizen', another Japanese concept, where there was a collective approach to creating a series of continuous improvements in our work. It used to be participative as we could actually voice our concerns and give constructive suggestions. The term 'quality circles' became a part of our work vocabulary and there was definitely an improvement in morale.

In all these concepts was the embodiment of enjoyment, productivity, a purpose, to move forward fruitfully.

As we speak of moving forward, we are reminded of the Tokyo Olympics 2020, which, braving many odds, came to a close with a modest medal haul for us in India and kudos for the Japanese for conducting such an event of mammoth proportions.

I recall a meeting and lunch with the Japanese Consul General, who had put up *koinobori*, carp streamers which had been prepared by his own staff. These colourful windsocks have carp patterns on paper or cloth and they flutter in the wind during Children's Day celebrations. The philosophy behind this is to wish children a bright future and hope that they grow up healthy and strong. The carp is a highly energetic fish and swims bravely upstream, fighting against cascades, and it is this determination that is used as a symbol of the upending of fortune and attaining of higher goals—something that the staging of the games signified with its modified motto, 'Faster, Higher, Stronger Together', to reflect a certain solidarity during the Covid pandemic.

And this serves as a representation of the **upstreaming of connectivity and positive communication** that we keep harping on in this book—**to swim against the lockdown stream we encountered and keep our heads above water, with clear thinking and creative solutions**.

5

Bandage: Setbacks as Springboards to Success

What's life without some large reverse?
You've failed! It couldn't get much worse
But setbacks make you count
To learn at forward fount
And treat rebuff as springboard for successes diverse

There is one thread of commonality that runs through the stories of people who have had immense success in their corporate lives, as authors, as individuals crawling out from the depths of despair. It's the word 'failure' and other attendant ones that spell rejection and rebuff.

Famous writers love to talk about the piles of rejection slips that they collected in their initial years and we know the much-repeated story of J.K. Rowling being rejected by 12 publishers before she found success with her *Harry Potter* series and sold 450 million copies. Jhumpa Lahiri faced her initial bouts of rejection before *The Interpreter of Maladies* was widely accepted. And even Chetan Bhagat was rejected by eight or ten publishers before his *Five Point Someone* became a bestseller. There's Amish Tripathi as well—who has given us a completely new genre of mythology-based creative fact-fiction and wasn't the immediate choice for publishers—admitting that he stopped counting after 20 rejections. Other bestselling authors like Jeffrey Archer were turned down by no less than 16 publishers.

All this is leading up to what this chapter will focus on—the setbacks that can actually become the fuel for success. To me, personally, failure seems to be something internal, something of a non-fulfilment on an individual's part, whereas rejection happens from the outside, unbeknownst to people, often through no fault of their own.

In the context of facing the challenges of life when rejections occur, a conversation with Ambi Parameswaran, a great adman and brand strategist, was a chance to know how setbacks can be counted as blessings in the long run. He has spent nearly 40 years in the industry and now creates his own deadlines, with writing books, consulting with brands, and teaching and mentoring.

In my earlier interactions with him at a conference, he was the one at the receiving end of the lessons which he had garnered from his clients, showing that a person of his stature was a learner who then applied the principles to his strategic thinking. This time, the meeting was a virtual one. I found through his new book *Sprint: Bouncing Back from Rejection*, how he made rejection and defeat become the springboard to turn around sagging careers, blunted aspirations and failing business models.

What I needed to know from him was how facing rejection could have its plus points. A telling observation from him—when his hour-long lecture to a group on leadership lessons did not get him a standing ovation but his ten-minute discourse on rejection did.

To begin with, he felt that all successful people, authors,

entrepreneurs, sportspersons, business executives, academics and scientists have had to face rejection. But the 'r-word' sends shivers down the spine of an average millennial. Perhaps they have had it easy till now or perhaps they think all successful people were plain lucky.

He was referring to the millennials as those born between the years 1985 and 2000, those who were working in organizations and had had a cushy time of it, with regular increments and promotions. A certain complacency would have set in. But then with Covid, a digital disruption happened, something they weren't prepared for. Startups went belly up. This is when they have had to wake up and be ready to face the downside, face rejection and take a leap of faith into uncharted territory.

'I believe luck somewhere plays a role in everything, but you cannot depend on luck. You should get over rejection and find a way around it. It is possible that the path you choose is a failure. You try again. You are enterprising, but not just lucky. You cannot wait for luck to strike. If you are sitting in a cave, you cannot expect something positive to come to you. You need resilience. There is a difference between enterprise and buying lottery tickets every day. Sure, divine interference or luck can happen, as do mentors who drift in at a crucial stage. But it is at the end of the day an effort at capitalizing on rejection and not letting it destroy our inner confidence.'

Such advice gains credence when this expert speaks of his own early rejections by Hindustan Lever Limited (HLL) and how these rejections got their providential due in his advertising career. 'It served as realignment or a redirection of energies in a new direction.' So, if in the end you get to land a career that is in sync with your abilities and passion, is it about luck in finding another path, or is it sheer guts and the ability to soldier on?

The latter, definitely. And something else called the power of redirection. Parameswaran was 'rejected' twice in his HLL interviews, but instead of recommitting to yet another job, he used the rejection to 'redirect' and put his energies in a new direction. This was the world of advertising which he stayed in, grew and contributed to hugely. From this very world, he gives us an insight into the advertising world's business pitching, saying that if any ad agency veteran tells you that their agency won every new business pitch they participated in, take it not with a pinch of salt, but with a ton of salt. Again, in the context of losing and winning, here's a tale of 'how a disastrous pitch led to some serious introspection and to a bigger win.'

It is the story of a car account. Hyundai was entering India and the agency Parameswaran worked for sent a pitch, along with several other agencies. They did not win the account and started soul-searching soon after. His advice, therefore—introspect after each rejection. They had lost the Hyundai pitch. Yet, they had lost the battle, not the war. So, when the new Tata Motors car was getting rave reviews in the media, before they could even invite agencies for a pitch, his agency FCB Ulka—which had set up a marketing communication case study competition with a leading business school—reached out to the potential client. In the end, they won the account and Tata Motors stayed with the agency for a long time.

One of the people, whom he recruited after making him wait for many moons, did his bit for this car account when he got the famous Indian cartoonist and painter Mario Miranda to do some sketches for sunshades that would go on the windshield of the Indica. The original cartoon actually went on to adorn the walls of the Director of the Passenger Vehicles Business Unit at Tata Motors.

Whenever we talk of failures, think of the multiple stories about Chinese billionaire Jack Ma, one of the richest people in the world, a philanthropist, and the creator of Alibaba, a go-to amazing e-commerce portal. An excerpt from his much-quoted speech at the World Economic Forum in Davos in 2015, published on YouTube titled *Jack Ma: I've Had Lots of Failures And Rejection*, goes thus:

> I've had lots of failures. I failed for funny things. I failed a key primary school test two times. I failed three times in middle school. I failed my university entrance exam. I applied for Harvard University ten times and got rejected for all ten applications. I was rejected by thirty different jobs. I even applied for a job at KFC when KFC came to China but I still got rejected. I think we have to get used to rejections. The most important thing is to never give up. We have to keep fighting and keep [improving] ourselves.

Let's not forget about the other reverses—his application to be a waiter, to join the police force, and 28 other jobs, all were rejected.

Rejections went even further, for when he got to his holy of holies—Silicon Valley—he was unable to convince them to fund Alibaba. The first three years turned out to be unprofitable and there came a time when he was not far from bankruptcy. Perhaps Ma has articulated these failures more often than others, but his successes have given a special shine to these setbacks and been a lodestar for scores of people.

He and others have used this much-touted Japanese proverb—'you fall down seven times and stand up eight'. It should remind most of us of our childhood when we dusted off our bruised knees and elbows, and restarted to run to the finish. To put the record straight, it is taken from a Japanese proverb 'Nana korobi ya oki', which captures the spirit of resilience. It was, incidentally, the title of a book by Japanese author Naoki Higashida who had severe autism.

While Ma's successes have far outweighed his failures, yet this flamboyant tech magnate got into trouble for his speech in Shanghai criticizing Chinese regulators after his Ant Group's IPO was suspended by stock exchanges. Soon after this, Ma lost more than half of his wealth.

Let us now go to an instance of 'redirection' when, in 2003, Arianna Huffington was running for the post of Governor in California against [Arnold] Schwarzenegger and opted out of it after a survey showed she would have garnered only two per cent votes. In 2005, she changed tack and track, used her communication style to rejig and went on to launch *Huffington Post*. If that was not enough, she sold *HuffPost* six years later to AOL for $315 million. This could be a message to people to either persist with what they are doing in the hope of a turn of fortunes, or to take a bylane of rejigged redirection.

The other aspect of a tangential 'redirection' is reinvention. We talk about it glibly, but even when you reach the top you should keep going, seems to be the message when Parameswaran gives us examples of Geet Sethi and Prakash Padukone, champions in their respective sports of billiards and badminton. Both these sporting legends went ahead and formed the Olympic Gold Quest (OGQ)—a programme of the Foundation for Promotion of Sports and Games. This non-profit organization has a great mission at its core—to support Indian athletes in winning Olympic gold medals.

The pandemic weighed down on the Tokyo Olympics. Originally scheduled to take place from 24 July to 9 August 2020, the event was postponed to 2021 on 24 March 2020 due to the global Covid pandemic, the first such instance in the history of the Olympic Games (in 1940, Tokyo Olympics were cancelled due to World War II). However, the event retained the Tokyo 2020 branding for marketing purposes.

Geet Sethi, a long-time friend, whose cue-sports excellence my sports journalist husband championed and which we both followed closely, and his remarkable eight world billiard titles which made India proud, held on to his belief that the games would happen, though likely with very strict protocols.

Sethi had this to say about the continuity of the process: 'The very nature and essence of sport and, more importantly, Olympic sport pre-supposes excellence at the highest level, conviction and continuity. In the past, we have seen the Olympics proceed despite wars and famines and even though this current pandemic is a massive disaster for mankind, my sense is that the Olympics will be held. The athletes continue to prepare with full gusto and with complete commitment to their training.'

At every stage of writing this book, I am blown away by the willingness of individuals like Geet Sethi, whom I have not been in touch with for a decade now, to readily offer their comment. He has always been a natty presence and his faith in an uncertain future, when he talked to us, made for rashers of hope. We too hold on to our beliefs in positivity, action, commitment—the hallmark of achievers.

6

Courage: Techniques of a Techtonic Mind

The new entrepreneur is the one full of zing
To produce the newest best-in-class thing
But the handholding's done
By the investor he has won
Who has mentored his growth from shoestring to bling

Statistics can be stepping stones, but there is also the stone-pelting that can come when they become outdated. Hence, we will not spout numbers but talk in generality about India's healthy startup ecosystem, looking at it from a global perspective. According to a reliable source, we hope to see an excess of 250 unicorns by 2025. Some of the IPOs were extremely successful and amazingly oversubscribed.

In 2023, the Economic Times Startup Awards saw a goldmine of talent thrown up, with the newspaper reaching out to more than 100 of the country's top entrepreneurs, investors, industry groups and other stakeholders to compile a list of the brightest entrepreneurial talent. B2B e-commerce startup OfBusiness won the 'Startup of the Year' award for building a profitable business at scale. Competition and commitment aplenty and the courage to go that extra mile to bootstrap, start up and sustain.

The deeper one delves into the eddies of the entrepreneurial world, the more one sees the flip side of the 'heads-I-win' coin. It is the face that builds those 1,000 ships, it is the hand that holds tight and guides the startup through muddy waters of uncertainty, and it is the 'mentorable' mind that ingests the courage to go forward.

The basic premise is that behind every successful entrepreneur, there is a venture capitalist who is equally in risk mitigation mode. They are in the swim together. The best endorsement of this could be gleaned from Saurabh Srivastava, who is one of the avowed architects of the IT industry in India, one of the most revered institutional builders acknowledged in India and globally, and the one person who can be credited with creating a vastly empowered entrepreneurial ecosystem in India.

This Padma Shri recipient, a doyen of entrepreneurship and angel/VC investments, in a detailed interview with this author, shared vital practical insights, where the mentorship element loomed large.

'You have to differentiate between a captain and a coach. That is the same difference between an investor and a founder. You are a coach as an investor. You should mentor, but you also have to let them run the company. You could lose your money down the line. So the best way to invest: write off that money in your mind. Help them get more money. Once you are an investor, you are a partner. You are not a bank giving a loan.'

Srivastava goes on to elaborate further: 'When an investor puts in money, it is equity. Fundamentally, when you are an investor, you become their partner. You have made many mistakes yourself, so now you help them avoid mistakes. You help them access technologies and see if you can add value.

The more value you add to your investment, the better is the chance of success.'

A recent example will serve to illustrate how pragmatically this philosophy has been put into action by someone who is the co-founder and chair of key institutions of modern India focused on entrepreneurship. Institutions like NASSCOM, the Indian Venture Capital Association, the Indian Angel Network (IAN), which is said to be the world's largest investor group with 100 portfolio companies, 400 investor members worldwide and seven chapters. The London chapter was launched by the former British PM David Cameron at 10 Downing Street in 2014.

The example we share is something that came about as a response in pandemic times. Srivastava was backing a team at IIT Kanpur for a while now. In fact, he is on the Incubation Board at IIT. When the team came up with a waterless cleaning product for solar panels, competing with a company in Israel, he was certainly keen on getting them funded. But he was in Delhi, and the team in Kanpur. There was an issue of scheduling. To meet their target and reach their destination, there was only one way—hopping on to an overnight bus. They were not ashamed to admit it, and that said something to Srivastava. Here was a team that was really passionate about what they were doing and could go the distance, literally, to achieve it. They got funded well.

That's not the end of their startup saga. Srivastava, who, as the chairman of The IndUS Entrepreneurs (TiE) Delhi-NCR and IAN Fund, is one of the leading investors in Nocca Robotics (an IIT Kanpur-backed startup), talks about the letter that came from Prime Minister Narendra Modi asking for help in dealing with the scarcity of ventilators in the country.

At that point, Srivastava and the Nocca team had understood that existing business models would not work, so he decided to re-engineer how a product would be made and formed a task force. He brought on board many more people who had wide experience in hardware product designs, people from healthcare and medtech industry, among others.

The task force started working on a high-quality, low-cost ventilator. Every day, for 100 days, everybody got on a zoom call for two hours, sometimes longer. And within 100 days, NOCCARC designed, developed and installed a world-class, ICU-level ventilator in hospitals. Creating a medical product and bringing it to the market takes at least two to three years! Today, NOCCARC has over 3,500 ventilators installed in leading hospitals. Pricing-wise, their ventilators are considerably lower in cost than those of their overseas competitors.

In my interactions with people who are leaders, mentors and individuals who are the acknowledged experts in their domain, what struck me was how down-to-earth their responses were. Saurabh Srivastava could have talked from his Olympian heights, but then there is his backstory, which reveals an entrepreneurial hunger all along and feeling the pulse of new business startups from the beginning.

According to Srivastava, 'Entrepreneurship and innovation is not one of the ways to go for India. It is the only way.' You have to let go, leave a cushy job (in his case, it was Tata Unisys, which together with TCS controlled 70 per cent of market share in IT), and then make your own company.

He founded IIS Infotech in 1989 which was acquired by a UK-based company FI Group in a multi-million dollar deal. In the early 2000s, it became Xansa. He co-founded

NASSCOM, an organization which has been instrumental in building the country's IT industry, helping Indian companies compete on the global stage. Then came the founding of The IndUS Entrepreneurs (TiE), followed by Infinity Venture Capital, which financed and supported startups till the time they were mature enough to attract bigger investments. With the last mentioned, he created twenty more companies that have changed the rules in their own way. India Bulls, India Games and Avendus Advisors got their early funding from Infinity.

As the lodestar for the whole entrepreneurship and innovation scenario, and a visionary who built a phenomenal ecosystem where millions of startups could be funded and flourish, we wanted to know what advice Srivastava would give newbies with Big Ideas as well as to those who could be losing their way and have failed to make an impact with their lack of vision, passion, preparedness and ability to do a perfect pitch.

In his opinion, when the pitching happens, there has to be clarity in communication—there should be a genuine ring to it. Simplicity is fundamental too. Authenticity and transparency are highly valued by the investor. There has to be a quality and rigour to their thinking and they should not make blind aspirational pitches. For spreadsheets do not blow away the investor.

Furthermore, it cannot be treated as a beauty contest, but more like a quiz. 'You can walk in packaged, which will get you the attention, but not the funding. There is this whole thing about form and substance. Form will get you the hearing, but the substance will get you the money. If you want an appointment, you should be articulate, but when you present you have to be precise, concise.'

You must not be overly glib. Don't try to snow the investors. It is not just about wearing a good suit and having the right diction. You cannot confuse this with communication. If you cannot communicate your idea in five minutes, you could easily lose the investor. The founder must pitch the statement of objectives with clarity and authenticity.

Even if there are twenty people doing something similar, you need to do something differently. Success is about how you approach the market. If you are taking something to the market where your competitors become your collaborators, the chance of success becomes better.

There can be no complacency about competition. If founders feel there is none, it is a cause for worry. The world is full of smart people, and they may have already discarded the idea you have, so there should be some soul-searching.

Srivastava gives the analogy of a music system when he talks about substance, but something that is not presented with style. 'A music system in the olden days had many components—a tape recorder and a turntable, as well as a tuner, an amplifier and speakers. If you had the world's best pieces but with third-rate speakers, then all that brilliance would come out sounding bad. A Bose system with cheap speakers would not work. So if you do not know how to put it across, it matters. With scientists, for instance, their work talks for them. But in the business world, if you cannot communicate, you are nowhere. Packaging is very important, too. It is imperative as well to be able to communicate what you are doing and who you are. Put in a team member who is articulate. Be well prepared, turn up on time. If you are authentic, it works. Prepare, but do not fake it.'

Another couple of factors: passion and humility, one being the absolute belief in their product and the other, how the team looks at the nuts and bolts of the bottom line.

Having made over 100 investments till now, Srivastava asserts that the entrepreneurs he supports must possess a great idea, offer a unique service, have a competitive edge, operate in a large and growing market, and take a well-thought-out approach to market entry.

Not all of them succeed.

Some companies succeed in the same space, others do not, and the difference lies in leadership. A good product, competitive differentiation and branding strategy are all necessary conditions to succeed, but not sufficient. A B-class team can make a hash of an A-class idea, but an A-class team will manage to build a business even with a B-class idea. In fact, anytime he got seduced by someone presenting a good business plan, if he was not comfortable with the founding team, every single one of them failed. It may have been the best technology put forward, but by the wrong people, those without the right value systems, no matter how sexy their product was.

Ultimately, he distinguishes the potentially successful entrepreneurs as those who want to do something different or something differently. The winners are the ones who take it to the market first and at an affordable price.

What does the future hold? It is the 20 per cent privileged population of India that should do something for the 80 per cent who are underprivileged. Having crossed many professional milestones in his life, Srivastava is now involved with many non-profit organizations. Like the NASSCOM Foundation, the community arm of the Indian software industry association.

Srivastava, as an éminence grise, sees large-scale changes kicking in through their initiatives. He has a pile of public service commitments and educational initiatives to take forward.

Mentors never rest but pave the way for the next in line to add to an enhanced startup ecosystem and are always accessible to give actionable advice. For those in the entrepreneurial stream, the tips given on these pages, put succinctly and simply by him, could provide some jump-up activation.

7

Curettage: The Wellness of Medical Conviviality

For wellness we swoon as illness spells doom
In times Covid-stricken when just negatives loom
There are healthcare frontliners
And surgeons who are heart-miners
They in combo give the populace optimism room

Reams and reams have been spun out by journalists, bloggers, self-appointed know-it-alls, in decoding medical terminology—from the Covid-affected and the vaccine sceptics to those paranoid about protocol. Yet, more than the pandemic, it was the disinformation that caused a canker in our psyche. But what about the doctors, surgeons, diagnosticians, health workers, Covid warriors—the ones who were the real players in the sickness scenario? Where, as the song goes, do they all belong?

Books that were prophetic erupted, and tomes that were meant as healing tools appeared too. But there is one which we found extraordinary in its scope, depth and scholarship and its pragmatism. Coming from the pen, rather than the scalpel of Dr Kunal Sarkar, a noted cardiac surgeon, *The Sickness of Health* is something that must be read, savoured in doses, as much for its historicity as for its current focus on healthcare.

At the heart of the matter is the fact that 'it is the will to live that forms the basis of the species to fight illnesses and injuries.'

I would term the reading of it as the Artichoke heart experience. My first experience of eating artichokes happened at my friends the Faulkners' vineyard Le Grand Cros in Provence, France. Each person was served one artichoke, looking for all the world like a green rose. You had to pull off one leaf at a time, dip the fleshy end in melted butter or a prepared sauce, grip the other end of the petal and scrape off the soft fleshy portion with your teeth.

A book like this was very much like the peeling away of an artichoke, as each leaf had meaning, each chapter pointing us to the historic background of medical colleges, of the state of healthcare, affordable or otherwise, medical tourism, doctors, whether they were to be seen as healers or predators, the Covid warriors, and much more.

Some of the unravelling was done through a heart-to-heart chat on the phone and mail-to-mail detailing during the difficult Covid times to understand how a surgeon had been reaching out, not just through the writing of a book, but much more to educate, demystify, tend to and give succour during the trying times of a pandemic, and how people like Dr Kunal Sarkar, one of the busiest surgeons in the city of Kolkata, set about tackling the problem, through action and by writing the book.

This chapter comes in the form of questions and answers—a change from our essayed format. It is akin to the artichoke petals that can be taken off one at a time and savoured.

Question 1: What compelled you to write *The Sickness of Health*? To bring greater awareness about the healthcare system and demystify it for the average reader? To give people a holistic picture through a historical perspective? To highlight the challenges of public–private partnership in healthcare in India—in the belief that it will gain traction with policymakers? What are your prescriptions for affordable healthcare? To do some shock therapy?

Answer 1: The news that Covid was spreading from China to Europe via Iran was initially met with denial in India, and we were amongst the many who also lived in the hope that it would blow over India. It was in January 2020 that we were shaken out of our denial with the first case being recorded on 30 January 2020. As we were bracing for the worst with a sense of facing the unknown, the dreaded lockdown was announced in March 2020. We, amongst many other clinicians, were suddenly engulfed with a sense of void. Routine work had abruptly come to a screeching halt. There were hectic discussions every day, going through the drills of what it might be like when we were flooded with cases. I was as confused and clueless as most of my colleagues. This is when I decided to plunge into an idea I had toyed with for long, to chronicle the journey of healthcare in India.

I have, after all, been very interested in the various healthcare systems in various countries. Returning to India after eleven years in the UK was a stark transition from a government-funded and administered structured system to a society where half the patients were lapsing into debt. A day in hospital cost more than their year's earning. The void of the lockdown was filled up with hours of amateur writing and background research.

Question 2: In the chapter 'Medicine and Media', you have laid out the pros and cons of media in wartime and peacetime.

Have you personally managed to use the media proactively, both digital and print, to get across your viewpoint? Can't audio, print, visual and cloud media be used to further your counselling ideas for information and assurance to people?

Answer 2: Doctors and hospitals have felt the need to communicate for the purposes of awareness and also to 'advertise' their domain expertise. The basic fact of prevention and management of common conditions needed to be spread to the community. It is only in the post-Independence period that common people had some access to medicine and surgery. They needed to be given some hope from the despair that every sickness meant impending death.

Some advertising was essential, but some of it was toxic as well. Since the 1980s, with the entry of the corporate sector in healthcare, commercial interests were high in the priority list. That heralded a flood of advertising campaigns and advertorials...the essential had morphed into the toxic.

Question 3: You have often talked of courage being the only medicine for Covid, which we have to defeat mentally and physically. Through many of your public speeches and TED talks, you have brought out not so much the work of the frontline workers, which is evident, but the resilience of people from the slums—Mumbai's Dharavi being a case in point and Kolkata's Belgachia. Is this your way of communicating positivity to people?

Answer 3: Courage is a part of the survival instinct. This was never more apparent than in these recent times when we were confronted with an unknown enemy, the first time in 120 years. The pride of the medical fraternity, who were able to fight successfully against most of the common ailments, had suddenly been reduced to helplessness. The common people never lost hope. They fought through breathlessness and fever, they were carrying patients to hospitals, ferrying oxygen cylinders to homes, feeding those whose livelihoods had melted away. These were soldiers in the forefront of the war for survival. It was the courage of the poor and the slum dwellers that was germane to India emerging from the calamity.

Question 4: Traditionally, doctors did not talk about their 'craft', and in fact were not supposed to advertise their operational skills. But do you find all this has changed because doctors feel that the patient has a right to be informed, to know details about illnesses and cures, and new methodologies? Are you responsible for changing the narrative with open, transparent communication?

Answer 4: In this era of information technology, with Google giving way to AI, information is readily available. But what about those who do not have access to digital avenues? After all, the internet penetration is less than 25 per cent. So, we cannot take anything for granted. We have to offer comprehensive and realistic counselling. In the world of private medical entities and their sense of sibling rivalry, there is a trend of one-upmanship and also trying to steal a march on our peers. This does not bear well for the profession.

Question 5: People turn to you as much for your medical sagacity as for your historical and literary allusions, your turn of phrase, all of which help in the ultimate process of striking the right chord with people. Do you believe that this is also an essential part of communication—the breaking down of the gobbledygook and the deconstructing of medical hyperbole into ways in which people can comprehend, relate, enjoy?

Answer 5: It is vital that we demystify the barrier of tough jargons. This has always been a daunting task. With medical discussions being quite popular in mainstream media and that too in the vernacular, it has helped matters. With Covid, there was an explosion of media conversations; this made it compelling for us to reach out to the millions of viewers in the simplest possible manner.

Question 6: You have praised many Southeast Asian nations for controlling the Covid pandemic in their countries. But you have talked about how India has lagged behind in its efforts. Reason?

Answer 6: India faltered in the initial stages of Covid management. Though 'health' is a state subject, the Centre assumed control via The Epidemic Diseases Act, 1897, which was rational. But there was a series of tentative actions.

a) Top of the list was a mistimed lockdown when the infections were at the lowest. As the first wave peaked and the country was limping back after a three-month lockdown, we were forced into lifting the suspension of life and living.

b) As the first wave was declining in October 2020, there was triumphalism all around. We did not notice the deadly delta variant and were caught off guard with the deadly second wave in April 2021. There was a rampant shortage of beds and oxygen.

c) Vaccination was deferred for two weeks on astrological grounds. The most baffling aspect was that through the

Covid struggle we never knew who was the Chief Epidemiologist leading 1.3 billion people.

d) Last but not least, WHO rubbished our claim of five lakh lives lost by suggesting that it was more than five times that estimate. Not good for Indian credibility.

However, it should also be noted that for both Covid and non-Covid diseases and illnesses, we have run the largest vaccination programmes in the world.

Question 7: In your own words, you are 'incorrigibly addicted to each and every detail of healthcare.' So what is your panacea for the scenario to bounce back? The intent of policymakers, administrators and bureaucrats—can they contribute to reviving the social and healthcare fabric of our country?

Answer 7: There are many weak spots in the fabric of Indian healthcare. More than 60 per cent expenditure on health was being done 'out of pocket'. The average for any other comparable country is 20 per cent. This has pushed millions into crippling indebtedness. Thanks to the health schemes, that deplorable statistic (of shame) is improving. Recent data suggests that it has come down to 40 per cent. We still have a long way to go. It is good to see that structured efforts are bearing fruit. At the same time, uptake of general health insurance is also improving. It is likely that Indian healthcare will end up resembling the US system with a mixture of general and government insurance.

Nevertheless, there have been significant achievements. Since Independence, the average life expectancy has increased from under 50 years to over 65 years. In a matter of five decades, we have reduced our maternal mortality rate and infant mortality rate to half of what these used to be. Every major tertiary specialty is practised with world-class outcomes. India is leading the way in pharmaceuticals and medical devices. Indian-made stents and advanced heart valves have a lion's share of the usage in Europe and the US.

Question 8: Although you have criticized the MBBS disappointments, the brain drain, the lower number of women coming into the medical profession, do you feel that the scenario can change? How? What could be the new motivations and dispensations?

Answer 8: There are certain basic features of medical education that are critical for the country.

First, doctors should be trained as a proportion of both population requirements and the infrastructure available. The WHO recommendation is a ratio of 1:1000. We were at 1:2000 about a decade back; now we are at 1:850! So, we have overshot the parity ratio. Secondly, with the viral proliferation of private medical colleges, of the 110,000 fresh medical graduates, 60 per cent are now from the private sector. Obviously, these seats come at a huge cost, eliminating the lower- and mid-class and indigent sections. The entrance exam benchmarks have been drastically lowered to take in those paying astronomical 'donations', sometimes more than a crore rupees for a seat.

India surely needs at least double the number of hospital beds. The accepted ratio is 2.5 per 1,000; we now have 0.5 per 1,000. So, we come to the crossroads of where are the doctors going to work?

India is entering a perilous decade of the oversupply of doctors having soft merit, with slow expansion in infrastructure.

This is sarcastically referred to as 'cash and carry' system of manufacturing doctors.

Question 9: Do you think India should ramp up its efforts in medical tourism? But is it possible in the current post-pandemic scenario? What an example Thailand has set with its Bumrungrad Hospital! Why are we so poor at marketing our facilities? For Bangladeshis, West Bengal should have been an entrepôt. Instead, patients veer to Thailand.

Answer 9: Kolkata hospitals depend largely on Bangladesh and the business share is less than 10 per cent. One has to remember that to be a healthcare destination, you have to be a preferred destination first! The urban profile and connectivity of Kolkata is low-key compared to that of our other urban peers.

Karnataka has 6,000 private hospitals while West Bengal has less than 700! Kolkata suffers in comparison to Singapore, which is a far more dazzling destination, with good medical infrastructure but also five times the cost. India is the only developing country where patients from higher income countries come for heart, joint and neurological surgeries, as well as organ transplants.

Question 10: On Doctors' Day, you had talked about how we lost 1,500 doctors to this 'war' and more lives than we did in the two years of our struggle for independence. You had to sound grim but at the end of the day, you have your positive streak. Therefore, is there a need, more than ever, to relentlessly and proactively communicate?

Answer 10: The sacrifice and selflessness with which doctors faced the pandemic were exemplary. The chivalry of the young interns and students, who were thrown before the lions during the second wave in 2021, is yet not acknowledged. Some of them who had never touched a patient before were now fighting a dreaded respiratory pandemic. The nurses and the supporting staff, more than 60 per cent of whom were young girls, were no less than a soldier in the Kargil Heights. Each 12-hour shift with the PPE suits would make them dehydrated and weak. They went on day after day.

We have never known how many nurses and supporting staff sacrificed themselves on the pyre of Covid. Shed a tear for them and their families. Those who survived have never had a health checkup since; they moved on from one shift to the next.

Question 11: Finally, has your debating avatar given a huge dimension to your persona, with people admiringly following your solid arguments as much as they follow your prescriptive talks?

Answer 11: My time in school has infused in me the passion for public speaking and being aware of history and relevant socio-economic affairs. I had a very cash-strapped youth, so school was both education and fun. Public speaking/debating has made it easier for me to reach out to people. I also have my social media platforms, which enable me to discuss issues outside of the medical precinct.

Bangla television has been a very effective platform. In the TV debates, I have not shirked away from giving a piece of my mind to the politicians. I admit this has mostly been received in the right spirit.

When we recall our debating days in school and thereafter in college, we must acknowledge the large debt we owe to the likes of Sudhangshu Dasgupta, N. Vishwanathan, Professor P. Lal, and of course our very own Kishore Bhimani. We learnt a lot from his speaking acumen and listening to his commentary was a lesson in language as much as it was an appreciation of cricket.

My debating colleagues and I reach out to schools across the states through the Calcutta Debating Circle, conducting debates and workshops for the young students. Regardless of the language—English, Bangla, Urdu, Hindi—the young ones are much better than what we were. The talent and intellect are all there... It is our duty to water the green shoots.

Positivity is key. Communication is the perpetual watchword.

8

Diplomage: Creating Coherence, Concord, Confluence

The language of diplomacy speaks with an ordained voice and form
The barriers more geo-politic, in keeping with all spelled out norm
But the universal language of music speak
Can these divides in euphonic ways tweak
To give voice to new areas of cultural cuneiform

Diplomatic moorings do not brook any full stops. Ambassador Nirupama Menon Rao, the former foreign secretary, has been in a life continuum beyond her four decade-long career in Indian diplomacy. From the moment I set eyes on this perfectly coiffeured woman in a vibrant Kanjeevaram saree, she held me spellbound with her effervescent personality, her approachability, and her quietly powerful demeanour. So this is what ambassadors are made of, I mused. Appearance, attitude, authenticity, amiability, academic acumen and something that she has come to signify post her illustrious career in diplomacy: ambidexterity.

Precisely what we bring to focus in this chapter where we look at how not to hang up our boots, or heels as it were, and how Rao first stepped into the world of academia immediately after retirement from active diplomatic service, and then with her deep and abiding love and passion for music, she set out to create the South Asian Symphony Foundation. She had always felt the need for a platform to promote dialogue, cultural synergy and friendly understanding among the youth of the region, resulting in the journey of promoting peace through greater cultural integration.

Our free-flowing fireside chat, organized by the Ladies Study Group, a prestigious organization that's been around for half a century, drew out some of the impulses that propelled Rao into the new venture. And of course, it is the connectivity and communicability in the toughest situations demonstrated by one of our ablest diplomats in the persona of Rao that completes the dynamic macro picture for us.

There are twin aspects that will find convergence in this chapter. One is the diplomacy of a getting-down-in-the-trenches kind, which spun off into some of the initiatives I would like to highlight here, and the other is the whole cultural diplomacy through the forming of the South Asian Symphony Orchestra that could be called a crowning point of a post-retirement career.

That the role of a diplomat goes well beyond handshakes, joint statements, and engaging in the highest circles could be seen in the numerous ambassadorial postings of Rao we have followed. For instance, as high commissioner of India to Sri Lanka, the political developments were tense and critical when Rao saw the assassination of the foreign minister Lakshman Kadirgamar and handled the fallout of the huge tsunami and personally oversaw the administering of relief operations for affected areas of Sri Lanka, including the war-torn North and East of the country.

After having worked in the Ministry of External Affairs for an unprecedented eight consecutive years (1984-92), with special focus on Sino-Indian ties, in 2006 Rao became India's first woman to be appointed as an ambassador to China. She expanded the Cultural Wing of the Embassy of India, transforming it into a hub of cultural activity, and set up the India China Business Forum. She was also there for the devastating Sichuan earthquake a few months before the Beijing Olympics, visiting the affected cities personally and ensuring the $5 million in relief coming from India.

When we look at her ambassadorial stint in the US, we find her playing a strong advocacy role for the bilateral relationship between the US and India. The Cultural Centre in Washington owes a lot to her pioneering efforts, first at acquiring the property and subsequently as a hub of high-profile cultural events. Her initiative found the inscribing of the Embassy residence in the register of historical (heritage) residences in the upscale Cleveland Park neighbourhood of the city.

Earlier, as India's foreign secretary, she was active in handling India's relations with its neighbours and with the US, Russia and Japan, besides multilateral issues including nuclear energy cooperation as well as climate change.

Rao's tenure as the first woman spokesperson for the MEA coincided with several significant events, including the July 2001 Agra Summit between India and Pakistan, the December 2001 attack on the Indian Parliament, and the subsequent standoff between India and Pakistan.

What we find interesting in our connectivity and communication imperatives that we are advocating in this book are the frequent live briefings for the print and electronic media. And even more significant, for someone who started the practice more than a decade ago, was the use of social media among government officers, when she made special efforts to augment and intensify the activities of the Public Diplomacy Division of the Ministry of External Affairs, increasing its outreach significantly.

Social media assumed more significance during the evacuation of Indians at the time of the 2011 Libyan crisis when she was commended for using her Twitter account (presently X) to regularly update the public about the evacuation, and also to respond to requests for help from stranded Indians in Libya. The X following today is a humungous 1.3 million and counting. It is all about positive connectivity and tweeting is just another arrow in her quiver.

So, from the peace-keeping overseer to the harbinger of peace through music, we now come to another facet of this able archer—the part that constitutes cultural diplomacy with the formation of the incredible concept of the orchestra. It is a huge tectonic shift and I dub it the art of the tangential, or refocusing your priorities in life. Having completed a hugely successful innings as a diplomat and then an educator in prestigious US universities, and keeping several balls in play writing books, a new melodic sequence has made a significant impact on the musical scenario of South Asia. When you are done with your key assignment in life, it is time to re-address your real passion and take it forward. That is precisely what Nirupama Rao, who has been a top ambassador and high-level strategic planner in the political arena, opted for. The change to an innate passion and the growing of it proactively.

And there is the bigger dispensation. Rao spells it out by saying how the need for a humanitarian agenda for the region built on closer people-to-people ties and citizen-driven cultural diplomacy is greater than ever. With Afghanistan, Pakistan, Nepal, Bangladesh, Bhutan, India, Sri Lanka and the Maldives making up South Asia in modern-day maps, Rao with her intense love for and involvement with music found the need to set up a platform 'to promote dialogue, cultural synergy and friendly understanding amongst the youth of the region.' She spelled it out further: 'Diplomacy is, at its essence, about people. We all have it within us to be "citizen diplomats", to reach out across borders and build bridges. The sturdiest bridge is the bridge of music. The love of music touches the very core of human existence, conquering divides, connecting diverse sets of people and nations, creating positive opportunities for human contact and communication, even among apparent adversaries.'

You have to see, experience, tune into and immerse yourself in the orchestral performance, which I did, to comprehend the magnitude of the movement. I call it musical diplomacy at its most pragmatic and prolific after witnessing the 65-musician-strong South Asian Symphony Orchestra (SASO) in Bengaluru, with the musicians forming a holistic connect for a 'region' that is Asia, but actually existing in a 'polyharmonic geography' in Rao's interpretation.

Appropriately named Chiragh, the orchestral movement is a true spark for opening up avenues for public diplomacy, designed as it is to 'promote peace building in the region: an Indian creation with a heart that is South Asian.' It is meant to 'craft a shared musical identity of the subcontinent of South Asia that is rich, composite, yet plural, helping the rest of the world view the region in a new light.'

The music that one experienced surely melted territorial

barriers, and in the process melded into a harmonic Peace Concert, which was titled 'From Gandhi to Beethoven—the Call to Freedom'. The concert—in celebration of 150 years of Mahatma Gandhi's birth anniversary—stood out for the presentation, an eclectically curated programme that gave the purists their favourite Beethoven concertos, but also knitted into its repertoire original compositions and regionally popular tunes, many of these numbers raga-based to create a euphonious whole. The musicians came from as far afield as Afghanistan, Nepal, Sri Lanka, Singapore, Thailand, Kazakhstan, the US, the UK and Germany, many constituting the South Asian diaspora, and of course different parts of India, in an orchestra that had the full complement of violins, violas, cellos, basses, flutes, oboes, clarinets, bassoons, horns, trumpets, trombones and percussion.

Why this emphasis on peace? In an interactive session and a mini-concert of selections from Rossini and Gluck, which I attended a day prior to the concert, you could see the diversity in a microcosm, listen to the pain of some of the musicians and understand how the political tensions, the conflicts in the South Asian region, and a huge amount of insularity have spurred on the whole idea of creating a movement like the South Asian Symphony Foundation. The larger goal: developing a 'humanitarian agenda for the region, built on closer people-to-people ties and citizen-driven cultural diplomacy.'

In talking of continuity and creativity in communicative techniques, which our book sets out to expostulate through its various chapters, this unique proposition of the Foundation, co-founded by Nirupama Rao and husband Sudhakar Rao, the former chief secretary of Karnataka, is one of immense proportions, spreading the message of regional cooperation, creating new music that is going beyond our shores, but is strongly rooted in our tradition.

Some of the stories of the musicians surely need a retelling here. While the conductor of the orchestra was a young Singaporean Alvin Arumugam, another conductor of the Afghan National Symphony Orchestra, Arson Fahim, a pianist, shared his tales of growing up in turbulent, war-torn Afghanistan. He had to overcome fundamentalists trying to silence their music, including that of an all-woman orchestral set-up called Zohra in Afghanistan. Interestingly, some of the hijab-clad women from Zohra also play in the SASO. The SASO is trying to find ways to reconnect with some of these musicians in Afghanistan or in the other countries where they have gone after the 2021 Taliban takeover.

The youngest is just thirteen, there's a flautist from the US Coast Guard (who played in uniform on the day of the concert), a cellist from Kazakhstan who leads the field at the Trivandrum Academy of Western Music, a musician who is a chartered engineer from Sri Lanka, and one from Nagaland, who started musical studies from the tender age of eight. All of them diverse, but consonant in their commitment.

One hastens to mention that there has never been a concept like this orchestra ever before. There was of course the West–Eastern Divan Orchestra founded in 1999, which had Arab and Israeli musicians from areas of conflict, and was formed by renowned musician and conductor Daniel Barenboim and equally celebrated scholar Edward Said, with the belief of improving relations in West Asia through music. But this one was born innately out of peace building in this region, and hopefully will overcome the underlying differences in a vast region like South Asia. Rao has enunciated it through her own album *Peace is My Dream*.

To capture in brief some of the highlights of the Peace Concert, the invocation 'Vaishnava Janato' by an Indian-American set the mood, followed by a Harmony Children's Chorus whose vast repertoire has seen them perform at Carnegie and raising funds for orphanages; the tapestry of traditional and popular works from the region in 'Hamsafar', a musical journey through South Asia; the Beethoven concertos with a pianist from Kerala and a musical tribute to Mahatma Gandhi by a 26-year-old Indian born in Verona. Bringing the curtains down on this eclectic concert was an encore that brought the best of our old film numbers into a dramatic fusion. Maintaining a delicate balance between youth renderings, invocation and classical, it was a mellifluous whole, so concordant, so complete.

The scenario of connectivity sees another completion when I rewind to my first chance meeting with Nirupama Rao. It was at the home of retired ambassador Sarvajit Chakravarti and his charming educator-writer-choreographer-singer wife Rupa, when they opened it up for a luncheon afternoon filled with poetry, music, discussion and an excellent culinary spread. This continued to be replicated regularly with formal invitations and diplomatic niceties observed, until the pandemic set artificial brakes to it all. But there has been no let-up in societal diplomacy as the couple continues a discerning upholding of culture and heritage. The foreword by Nirupama Rao in Chakravarti's book titled *Pilgrimage* is something that the author acknowledged as 'the ultimate fruition of realizing that mine was a life well spent'.

Rao's own latest book is titled *The Fractured Himalaya: India, Tibet, China 1949–1962*. It is a diplomatic and political history of the relations between India and China in the crucial decade leading to the border-related conflict of 1962.

The erudition and educative aspects reflect a person of deep learning. We need to live by what she had said at the convocation ceremony at a university about aiming 'at becoming the gold standard in open governance, enshrining respect for human rights, internalizing respect for the history that makes us what we are, a diverse and plural society, and a rejection of the closed mind.'

We hope mega movements like SASO will see more workshops, master classes and enhanced initiatives in creating and composing new work, the adding of instruments, upping of citizen support, voluntary donations and fanning of corporate intent so that talent can develop and get an international lift. 'The interest of a global audience in our country will only deepen,' says Rao, 'if we are seen as reaching out and speaking a global language of music.'

Ambassador Rao looks to a cultural renaissance for India which is rooted in the culture of humanism. 'Music provides humanism with an ideal vehicle; it is a natural vector for giving voice to the unknown, unsung men and women who escape the attention of the more privileged amongst us.'

The linkages are ongoing. In 2021, in a virtual performance honouring former President Joe Biden and Vice President Kamala Harris, the South Asian Symphony Orchestra was part of the musical offering represented by a Sri Lankan-American musician. The outreach of music is a true measure of cultural diplomacy.

9

Engage: Riding the Radio Waves of Connectivity

You see me not, but you hear me still
I'm the voice that brings you thrill
Through engagement and connect
To make you want to reflect
And be your balm, your calm, your vitamin pill

The signature tune of All India Radio was our waker-upper in our teenage, when the ABC of our lives spelled audio-bioscope-chatter, with no handheld devices to interfere with our direct communication airwaves, and no bright computer screens blinding our focus. Hearing was all-important. The haunting melody, repetitive in its intent but resonant in tearing at the heartstrings, had been composed by the most unlikely of people, the Czech-Jewish composer Walter Kaufmann, and the tune was based on Raga Shivaranjini. This Jewish refugee was to become the director of music at AIR (1937–46) and immerse himself in understanding Indian classical music.

Radio was a major hero of our homes, so this tune became part of our psyche.

Did radio ever go away? Not for me, not for the new era of aural audiences who are enjoying brand new ways of connecting and interacting.

Growing up with radio was initially a very personal affair. Bulbul Sarkar, known for her dulcet tones and her impeccable accent as Auntie Bulbul in *Calling All Children* and for producing Western music at All India Radio Calcutta, was an actual aunt of mine. Interestingly enough, she too had a Jewish connection as she learnt voice modulation for radio and piano from a Jewish lady who had fled from Vienna.

From her we learnt the finer nuances of Western classical music, heard the concerts of famous visiting musicians who would come to New Empire—the likes of Yehudi Menuhin and Benjamin Britten; but most of all, we were impressed with her series of illustrated talks done in conversation with Satyajit Ray: *What Beethoven Means To Me, Music I Live By, Music In My Films*.

Thus, it was a natural thing to be at AIR doing programmes for the youth and receiving minuscule cheques of ₹10 and ₹15 so that when we got our first cheques for Doordarshan's newsreading, ₹75 seemed so handsome! Radio could never get out of one's system, as a monthly programme for Radio South Africa saw one doing a whole women's hour 'Letters from Calcutta' for listeners in faraway Cape Town, using very basic technology.

As users of radio, we had the guilty moments of tucking transistors away in office drawers to listen to the running commentary, but also actually gained some learnings from the Rabindra Sangeet lessons by Pankaj Mullick, got au fait with Western pop, jazz and blues through lunchtime variety, and could never ever leave the haunting Mahalaya *stotra*s (hymns and prayers) of Birendra Krishna Bhadra. It was Bhadra who first heard my husband's voice covering the 1971 war following which he urged Kishore to try his hand at cricket commentary, which eventually started off a lifelong career. And then there was our son who was so wound up about doing his *Good Morning Calcutta* series when FM radio first started that the non-morning person in him would see him motivated to jump out of bed, carry his pile of CDs and do a supercharged programme where celebs would drop in for good measure.

We developed our favourite commentators and newsreaders: you knew them by their accents, the lilt of their voices, and the style of presentation, so it did not matter that you could not see them. And for sheer continuous entertainment through the hit songs from Hindi films, there was Radio Ceylon with *Binaca Geetmala*, from the fifties to the eighties. The presentation by Ameen Sayani used to be electric.

Things changed. Our tastes altered. The idiot box intruded. When audio got its visual overlay with television dominating our lives, radio took a little bit of a back seat, but was to quickly resurface when FM channels became the flavour of the times. So it was the frequency modulation that made radio come right back with the privatization of FM broadcasting giving a new kick-start in the 2000s when the sound of music got enhanced, and the quality of programming took on fresh approaches. While AIR broadcasts in 23 languages and 146 dialects, and reaches out to more than 100 countries through its programmes by the External Services Division, FM radio is now seeing its own clutch of successes with over 200 stations and growing listenerships. Radio's direction is changing with the altered needs of its diverse audience.

I recall my time at the University of Georgia when sports broadcasting on radio was peaking. The year was 1965 and the football coach of the university, Vince Dooley, was thinking of going to another institution. The team of Radio WSB went ahead and recorded a song 'Won't You Come Home Vince Dooley'. He stayed on in Georgia.

Valour stories abound among the radio waves, and so we share some about one of our very own RJs in Kolkata, Jimmy Tangree. The city has several well-heeled FM stations in English and the vernacular, and it would take reams to write about these anchors and their following. We focused on Tangree of 91.9 Friends FM as someone whom we have seen grow from being a DJ at Calcutta Swimming Club, playing music rather than talking, to becoming the popular chatterbox RJ that he is today. To him, 'We are not just talking to people on air, but we are engaging and connecting and making a difference, making positivity, creating happiness in these pandemic times.'

What were some of these acts of kindness and happiness?

With his *Direct Dil Se* carrying on late into the night, there are unreal situations that an RJ like him encounters. How to deal with a razor's edge situation when a person is about to end his life and proclaims this on air? Tangree kept asking him a lot of questions and spoke to him reassuringly, keeping up the patter for a good fourteen minutes, before convincing him to get off the ledge and go back to his room. They have become good friends and radio gave that person a new life.

Romance has also been tackled with profound questions asked of a girl who was apprehensive about letting the object of her romantic gaze know how she felt. After forty-five minutes of friendly advice from our RJ, she called the guy to the terrace, blurted out that she wanted him to be her life partner, and they were of course united, with the follow-up story coming from Tangree that they are parents to two children today. The chiding helped.

Friends FM, in fact, launched its podcast site www.friendsdigital.com in May 2023 that gives listeners the opportunity to hear stories in 11 different genres, many of them based on true events. Radio is truly diversifying and inclusive.

So we come to an RJ who was a popular presenter on Radio Mirchi with *Dil Chahta Hai* and then with *Coffee House Classics*. She also headed Red FM in the east and was involved with Aamar FM as well. Roopsha Dasguupta did all this in various languages but finally came to accept the draw of the digital with her startup Oopsroops, which provides 360-degree brand and creative integration solutions for domestic and international clients. It aims to create budget-friendly and impactful content with its weekly shows *Joy of Life* and *MOTIVate*. And then there are her Friday podcasts.

For someone who has interviewed outstanding luminaries from Nobel Laureate Amartya Sen, Oscar-winner A.R. Rahman and superstar Amitabh Bachchan, to leading cricketers and singers like Asha Bhonsle, topped up by the last concert of the late Manna De at Coffee House Kolkata, Dasguupta's digital *ADDA-AAH* for the Bengali news portal *The Wall* is the first live web chat show of West Bengal.

What is this new webcasting all about? Is it advice being doled out or entertainment or both? For someone who had been called the last generation of blue-blooded radio professionals, her switching to podcasts showed that this was the way forward. Her husband gifted her a state-of-the-art microphone for a home set-up, which gave her the luxury of whatever she wanted to do. Her ten episodes on her mother's stories got plenty of shared stories and her Friday *Tarader Thhikanay Chhithhi Lekho* dealt with grief management.

The world of podcasts is expanding so fast that we are totally spoiled for choice, and according to a PWC 2020 report, India has the third-largest podcast listening market in the world with 57.6 million monthly listeners.

The bouquet of offerings covers ever so many passions of people, from the spiritual and motivational podcasts to those that focus on key issues of concern through *On the Contrary*, *Kahani Suno* that revisits the classic stories written by Jaishankar Prasad and Munshi Premchand, a bloodcurdling crime series, and a bilingual food show, among others.

Spotify, JioSaavn and Gaana have diversified their podcast offerings. So you could have your share from TED Talks, or tune in to Jaya Row's *Gita for the Young and Restless*, which, as the name suggests, delves into different aspects of life and attempts to provide solutions to contemporary problems, rather than being a high-handed discourse on scriptures.

If academic lectures and inspirational talks aren't your cup of tea, there's no dearth of options on the internet—from *Indian Noire*, a gritty crime thriller hosted by a gynaecologist, and *The Musafir Stories–India Travel Podcast*, to *Maed in India* if you have an ear for music, and *Stuff You Missed in History Class*, among others.

In a way, we are back to radio but in a different manner. You get it on the internet and it can be downloaded and saved and listened to at any time. Radio will continue to be the connecter in the main, engaging you, enticing you to react and empathizing with you whenever necessary. Actually, it never went away.

10

Envisage: Clickbait in the Age of Influencers

The spheres of influence have acquired new parlance
Where the consumer is pulled in at one clickbait glance
Forget the old ways
As the internet gaze
Makes the brand experts leave nothing to traditional chance

Influencer marketing is growing in billions of dollars, and the influencers are making a luxurious living as spokespeople for their own ideas and for those clients whom they represent. So, the contemporary consumer is just a clickbait away! And the influencer is not the wife or child in the family anymore, but the one who straddles the internet waves. The era of the social influencer is the here and now thing, with branding of products divorcing the traditional approaches for the power of mouth to reach millions through a single tweeted endorsement.

Influencing you into believing in and subsequently buying into a product has reached a different stratosphere and like it or not, but even the dyed-in-the-wool marketing specialists are using the power of the pretty young thing who has gained credibility as a social influencer with millions of followers. Oh yes, it is women who appear to dominate this space. As demographic statistics reveal, more than three-fourths of influencers who are creators of sponsored posts on Instagram are women. The total number of daily active Instagram users is a mind-boggling 500 million.

For those of us who have been grouted in the once-upon-a-time approaches of advertising, marketing and public relations communication, it is like getting on to Aladdin's magic carpet and soaring into digital space which is heady with numbers and rich with promises of reaching your target.

To make some real-time sense of it all, we approached one of the new-age influencer services agencies called Qoruz. Run by Aditya Gurwara, it empowers content creators with the necessary tools and guides to excel in building great influence.

So, the marketing trends, as seen by Gurwara, are the strengthened brand–influencer relationships, the tracking of actual sales from interactions with influencers and a focus on their performance, spotlighting the audience of the influencer to get the feel of the demographics and to have a check on brand–influencer fit, and looking at an outreach towards strategizing for targeting Tier 2 and Tier 3 markets with a greater focus on regional and vernacular. He feels that today's consumers go by the opinions of their friends or those whom they can relate to. And in that context, he agrees with Prasad Shejale of Logicserve Digital who says that a large swathe of consumers would put more faith in a social influencer than in traditional advertising or endorsements by celebrities.

It is impossible to come to terms with some of the number crunching that takes place. There are as many as 500,000 influencers, with a minimum of 50,000 to 60,000 followers each. Numbers that keep growing daily. As for their earnings, we learn from Gurwara that 21-year-olds are banking

₹30 lakh to ₹40 lakh a month. The influencers who have become highly sought after, quirky though many of them may be, charge ₹40 lakh for a single video.

Actor Sonu Sood, described also as a film producer, model, humanitarian and philanthropist, charges ₹20 lakh for an Instagram post. A single post of his reaches out to three to four million people. His popularity can be gauged from the fact that one fan cycled 1,200 kilometres just to meet him.

Actress Disha Patani has over 61 million followers. People remember her for her role in *M.S. Dhoni: The Untold Story* and a Chinese action-comedy *Kung Fu Yoga*, which is said to be amongst the highest-grossing Chinese films of all time. The numbers for other top-drawer actors are said to be even more massive.

But leave aside these celebs, it is the individual influencer, says Gurwara, who controls both content and distribution. The company using their services just does the payout, possibly from marketing budgets, and leaves the rest to attract eyeballs that translate into sales.

Then there are individuals who have reached humungous followers and subscribers in a space they have carved out for themselves. An example is 25-year-old Ajey Nagar who goes by the name CarryMinati. He has over 45 million subscribers on YouTube and 22 million followers on Instagram, more than 3 million followers on X (formerly Twitter), and over 2 million on Facebook (FB). And earns about ₹4 crore a year. The numbers change daily. It is his short videos made for the web that have a connect with millennials. And he has made a fine art of roasting without crossing limits.

To focus again on the brand-audience-influencer context, it is analytics that play a critical role. Agencies that leverage influencer marketing have large databases which can be used to have pinpointed bespoke solutions for clients. The influencers inhabit spaces like health, tech, fashion, food, lifestyle and sport, and use Instagram, Facebook or other digital media platforms. The agency makes sure that the audience which the influencers have matches the branding targets of their clients.

The true responsibility lies with influencer marketing agencies. They research into the audience that influencers have, to be able to absorb the finer points of demographics, and most of all, to see whether there can be a true merging of the influencer's mission and the vision of the brand. The analytics is also to ensure whether influencers are on the case of other competitive brands. It isn't all big-city-oriented but also takes into account vernacular sensibilities and townships where the reach could be more impactful.

The ecosystem has truly changed drastically. It isn't just about sourcing influencers. There is a larger science to the process. There are, for instance, the Advertising Standards Council of India guidelines that kick in to ensure that there is no conflict of interest, that content is above board, and to get influencers to reveal that they are actually promoting a product as an advertisement and not merely endorsing it personally. This ensures that there is transparency in the whole system.

These agencies also organize the pooling of micro-influencers and then connect these influencers with brands who are looking for image enhancement online. They also make sure of the veracity of the influencer's followers—the fact that they are real and not robots. They also help the brands craft their campaigns and ensure the eventual post is in line with that vision.

The internet has given immense power to influencers to become creators. From zero beginnings, and sometimes only basic education, an influencer commands large sums of money for a single tweet, because of his or her tremendous reach. There are phone brands which pay ₹15 lakh, Gurwara estimates, to speak about their product, uploading videos, perhaps a couple of times a week. There are also extra charges for exclusivity of promoting a product. But there can be no brand-bashing for sure!

A couple of examples will show the journey, the influence and the popularity of those who went into the online space at a time when such content creation and reach were unheard of. Take Masoom Minawala who is in the fashion space. She started ten years ago, and now she is recognized among leading women entrepreneurs worldwide by HSBC. She was also featured on CNN's 20 under 40 list. Importantly, she has collaborated with luxury fashion houses like Louis Vuitton, Dior and Bvlgari, as well as brands like Estée Lauder, Samsung, BMW and Airbnb, represented India at the Cannes Film Festival red carpet, and set up a fashion e-commerce platform catering to millennial women in India.

The story has continuity to it in the form of Minawala actually extending her expertise to help other women by highlighting women-led businesses and unique Indian designers through initiatives like Empowher and #SupportIndianDesigners. With Empowher, she hopes to create a space for working women and entrepreneurs to be able to openly talk about the problems and obstacles they face at the workplace.

And now let's get truly desi with *Social Samosa*! We spoke with Hitesh Rajwani who heads *Social Samosa*—a leading social media publishing website specializing in advertising and social media communication. It is followed by brand leaders, agency professionals, and of course social media enthusiasts.

Guess what? They also run the aptly named *Social Ketchup*, their influencer marketing arm, which features a well-illustrated and content-rich online publication. Having explored several issues, we found it packed with the latest trends and insightful stories related to social media. It also includes reviews of major campaigns, case studies and expert commentary from industry professionals. One of the editions we browsed through was a 60-page 'Pride Special', featuring in-depth interviews with LGBTQIA+ community members.

Social Samosa has enabled the industry with information symmetry and best practice benchmarking. The network promotes and facilitates data-driven digital marketing and lays stress on content marketing and devising digital intellectual properties. Over the years, the Social Samosa network has built and empowered an ecosystem where brands, agencies, creators and local businesses learn from the shared knowledge base and work towards developing a thriving industry

Rajwani, who is an MBA from Symbiosis, is the avowed expert in digital marketing strategy, brand management and experiential marketing. As a self-motivated entrepreneur, he has co-founded a couple of ventures in the space of digital content and propounded the theory of 'The Social Moment of Truth'. His areas of interest include social commerce, digital intellectual properties and hyperlocal commerce. His passion for building digital IPs has propelled him to build concrete industry mandates and platforms. He has been a speaker and panellist at industry forums like CII Kolkata and NASSCOM

CSR Conference Delhi, and a jury member at Inkspell Drivers of Digital Awards, exchange4media, IDMA and Indigo 6E Appsters. Over the years, he has consulted and trained small medium businesses regarding their social media marketing strategy. His varied exposure is testimony to a wide array of skills that range across marketing, communications and business development.

He also led us to track the stories of some of the popular influencers who have made the cut. One of them is totally rooted in comedy.

Prajakta Koli feels that she prefers to go beyond travel, fashion, DIY, cooking and tech content to focus on the humorous approach. With seven million YouTube subscribers, and a team of writers to boot, it seems to be a great space for a young woman who has just touched thirty to be in. She is best known for her comedy videos on her channel MostlySane. Earnings? Heavens! Her published net worth is ₹18 crore and her monthly income from YouTube is around ₹40 lakh and annual income ₹4 crore. She has become a popular figure on the screen with a Netflix India series, *Mismatched*, where she has a lead role; this is in addition to her debut feature film *Jugjugg Jeeyo*, a murder mystery *Neeyat*, and many others.

Prajakta was part of Forbes India 30 Under 30 and Entrepreneur India's 35 Under 35 list for 2019 and Outlook Business's Women of Worth, among many other such accolades. She attended the prestigious World Economic Forum held at Davos where she participated in discussions on climate change, social justice and global healthcare. She was also part of important discussions with the the National Commission for Women where Netflix hosted a special event on the role of entertainment and media in empowering women.

From being the whacky MostlySane to reaching international fora with a purpose is just what we advocate as the Presence Perfect factor in communication.

Another YouTuber and content creator, Niharika N.M. has to her credit millions of followers, and the fact that she got to the US just before lockdown was slapped on, and she had to deal with stressful situations, made her dream up the creation of content as a creative outlet. Her journey has become the topic of a case study at Chapman University in California, where she did her MBA. Her specialization? Thirty-second grounded videos that people can relate to because of everyday events that are woven in with expressions that reflect the South Indian way of life.

According to a 2022 *Forbes* article, the Los Angeles-based Indian comedian and content creator had over three million Instagram followers and over 700,000 YouTube subscribers. Her video 'Living Alone 101' went viral on Instagram and hit 14 million views in just under 15 days. Another video titled 'One Way Street It Is' hit 10 million views within a week. She has partnered with Netflix and Amazon Prime India and worked with brands like BYJU's and OPPO. She has won several awards and recognitions including Best Entertainment Influencer at the Impact Digital Influencers Awards and Blogger/Creator of the Year 2021 at the Women Disruptors Awards 2021 held by Adgully. She was selected by YouTube as one of the global ambassadors for the Creators for Change programme.

Many of the figures are quoted after our conversations with influencer marketing experts. But some of them are approximations, and it is just that they have been used here to show the big-league picture.

The language of communication for the influencer is now swerving to the regional where localized content makes for greater acceptability among audiences who can get content in their local languages. Affording a greater chance for micro-influencers to come forward and speak in a credible tongue. The style, though, has to be smart, savvy, sassy and swift if you are to make the immediate impact and the quick bucks that also go with connectivity through YouTube, Instagram and LinkedIn. Presentations are becoming more down to earth and marketers are lapping up the grounded connect to help their brands grow.

11

Encourage: Mentoring Mindspace to Munificent Wealth-Share

There are those who lead from the front, at business they are true ace Mentoring and building businesses that carry a human face
It is in their gifts of giving
And the sharing of their wealth for the living
That makes the philanthropy get a case for new base

One of the areas that corporates have been impelled to do by law is their CSR initiatives. Many do their two per cent as a token appeasement of corporate conscience. Increasingly, though, others have larger plans mapped out in community resource building and yet others, overawed by the likes of an Azim Premji giving away huge percentages of his personal wealth, loosen up their purse strings for the greater good. And for some, the lodestar is the manner in which the Bill and Melinda Gates Foundation has been hugely impactful in India.

In the course of reaching out to business heads, startup specialists and personages who have been making a difference in their fields, I found in Subroto Bagchi a visionary leader whose philosophy and progression illustrate a combination of growth and giving, of risk-taking and re-invention, and a values-driven approach to work life. Thus, it is that our chapter on the sharing of wisdom and wealth focuses not just on the mentoring, the networking that we have talked of in the other parts of the book, but also the point at which profits and wealth amassed are shared, distributed and used in non-profit ventures.

But there are some, like Bagchi, who have grown a company that has factored in the philanthropic oeuvre from the initial stages and not as an adjunct. In his own words, he helmed a company, Mindtree, which went beyond being just another software services company, as it would be pitched at doing 'aspirational work, a company that would create shared wealth and one that would have a social conscience'.

It is interesting to go back to Bagchi's journey to share the earlier setbacks of his career. 'Mindtree was conceptualized in mid-1998 when I found myself caught between two contending forces. I had made a wrong career decision and had left Wipro. I could blame circumstances but it was I who was responsible in the first place to have glossed over things while making the choice. I knew I had to move out. At the same time, there was a massive opportunity unfolding before me. The Y2K problem was a huge opportunity before the Indian software companies because for the first time, the legitimacy of doing large-scale work from India was getting accepted by the corner office of Fortune 500 companies. Yet, Y2K wasn't what the big deal was for me. A few of my co-founders and I saw big opportunities coming up in telecom and e-commerce. Thus, on one side, I had a wrong job move and on the other hand, a huge opportunity, albeit risky and uncertain. It was alluring. Then came the hard question: why should we start yet another software services company?'

He goes on, 'Getting together a group of like-minded co-founders wasn't difficult as I had my eyes set on them for a long time; I admired them as professionals and knew that there would be value-match, ahead of just shared vision. Values must override vision when one makes a monumental decision whose implications would be beyond what the eye sees.'

Another key factor worked in his favour where he set out to do work that would deliver outstanding value to customers, create shared wealth and in the process, build a business with a human face. As a first-generation entrepreneur, he talks with humility about being born to lower middle-class parents and going to vernacular schools, which probably made him stay rooted. 'I was deeply aware of life and living beyond the bubble. I never lost sight of it. While the job of business is largely business, I also saw how people like Azim Premji, Narayan Murthy and his co-founders were using business as a force of change. Thus, it wasn't difficult for me to understand the larger purpose of business—it is *larger* prosperity. Then I realized another thing and this had to do with the writer in me. And that I was capable of "humanizing" business as a narrative. Once I realized that, I think I could create a space for myself from which putting a human face on business was easy.'

Structuring a company of its proportions became a story of 'collective leadership'. While he facilitated the process of creating the mission, vision, values and the brand and was the face of these ideas, 'behind it all was a rare division of labour between the members of the top management that gave each other space, practised egoless work and made way for the best person for any job.'

'While I was doing these, someone else was getting

business, managing investors, creating governance processes and delivering the code. These were as critical as the work I did and founders who ran these engines were the best you could imagine. The arrangement worked like magic for the first ten years of the company which were the defining years.'

He even went so far as to move to the US 'to keep the flock together' as differences and cross-cultural issues cropped up with varied gene pools of the co-founders. The key was to sense it and 'respond before you get under the wave and that is what made me to shut shop in Bengaluru and move to the US in 2000.'

We often wondered at the unique designation of 'gardener' that Bagchi had adopted. The idea was not quirky at all as he believes that it came from the realization that the top 100 Mindtree minds must be groomed for bigger things. 'This would need paying individual attention as against sheep dipping them in leadership development. The idea of providing individual attention to a group of 100 high-performance leaders took us to the metaphor of a gardener. A farmer massifies the well-being of her crop. In contrast, a gardener must know each tree individually, recognize its unique needs and raise it as if it is the only tree in the garden. This needed total attention from someone senior and I opted for it. We had a unique process that was partly structured and partly unstructured so that we could make it work for each leader differently.'

As for the impulses and qualities needed to steer his enterprise, the Bagchi philosophy which should find resonance with people is when he talks of 'resilience ahead of winning and an abundance of mindset too.' He says, 'Understand the idea of instrumentality. I am not the centre of the universe.

Even the universe is not the centre of anything. Have urgency in everything you do, do it well, do it for everyone, and do it without compromising the means for the end. We need people who not only do the right thing but do it the right way. Values of the boardroom and values of the home are the same. You do not become a first-rate boss and a third-rate spouse at the same time. Life does not suffer that contradiction even as you may suffer the illusion.'

The measure of a person's progression is when they can go back to their roots with a new vision and visitation. The chief minister of Odisha invited Bagchi to come back to his state of origin by appointing him chairman of the Odisha Skill Development Authority. If Bagchi had not built his reputation one day at a time with four decades of work in the IT industry, maybe it would not have led up to the moment. 'Shri Naveen Patnaik made a phone call asking me to come. Life is that. Even as we do not see how the links in the chain hold. Yet the crossover to public life has been like getting off from one spacecraft and boarding another, each traversing what sometimes look like parallel universes. When you look at the larger issues on the ground, you see the development challenges confronting a country like ours, you realize how much of a bubble many of us live in. As for the sheer joy of working in public life, I would not trade the last seven years for the first forty years of my professional success in the private sector.'

To top it all and go back to our original premise about philanthropy, we find Bagchi and his author-wife Susmita Bagchi coming forward to donate ₹370 crore towards a cancer hospital and palliative care centre in Odisha, from their personal wealth. Additionally, they part-funded the Bagchi-

Parthasarathy Hospital at IISc, Bengaluru, at ₹212.5 crore to set up a postgraduate medical college and an 800-bed multispeciality hospital at its Bengaluru campus.

It is not often that we get to know first-hand the impetus that has propelled such a philanthropic gesture. Bagchi throws considerable light on this: 'When we saw the wealth coming our way, it made us deeply question our own selves. How much is enough? What part is truly ours? What is the burden of responsibility that must come from affluence? That is when we did some sense-making along with our two daughters and made a family decision that the bigger chunk of the money must go to serve public good, and that, ideally, must happen in our lifetime. It isn't easy to spend money in India, that is why a lot of people with money do not know how to engage. It is very different in other parts of the world. To find a cause, get the right partner, have the right governance model, and then combine all that with the desire to detach oneself from the money make it a big challenge.'

He had ticked all the boxes in my book—great visibility in the media and on television, reaching out with important messages on the pandemic and on entrepreneurship. Did it require him to be always at the ready? Because this is what we are propounding in *Presence Perfect!*—being ahead of the game, having your finger on the trigger, being alert to immediate issues and tackling them head-on. 'You must be always ready,' he says. 'The train stops only for a few seconds. Doors open and close in the blink of an eye. You do not know when the next train would arrive and on which platform.'

As the author of bestsellers like *Go Kiss the World*, a book that I had a chance to interact with him about when it was released in Kolkata, the main chord that he strikes is the simplicity and depth of messages, told linearly, in story form. But there was another book, *The Professional*, which needs iteration here, in that it talks of the ethics of being a professional, the codes of conduct that must exist if clients, customers and employees can trust the prescriptive advice doled out.

Hence, we continue to seek out tech innovator, mentor and public figure Bagchi, who has now moved on from the Skill Development Authority to being appointed chief advisor to the Odisha government for institutional capacity building across all civil service training institutions of the state functioning in the rank of a cabinet minister.

For the need of the hour is a continuum of creative thought, communicative action and a big leap forward in tomorrow's growth agenda.

12

Homage: Don't Walk Alone! Mentors Can Change Mindsets

The mentor's the one with the brains and big heart
As the mentee wants mainly to get a headstart
There's no dakshina charge
As he floats hopeful barge
For the shishya who must then make a play for rampart

Going it alone is no longer an option. The startup ecosystem is crying out for the entrepreneur to hitch her wagon to a mentor whose experience, credibility and, naturally, a willingness to help could become a game changer.

Many of us have prided ourselves on working for multinationals. We loved the largesse of these behemoths, the idea of their far-reaching empires, and the ability for us, individually, to connect with co-executives across continents. Big was synonymous with beautiful. But the new narrative shifted—from large corporations to an introspective, entrepreneurial one. The 'Start-up India, Stand up India' mantra is an example of the *atmanirbhar,* or self-reliant, stance that a section of people are warming up to. The self-reliance is, partly, a signal for 'Make in India' and 'Make for India', but it is also a call for entrepreneurs to pursue their Big Idea.

It is in this environment that mentorship gives a fillip to

the newbie, the one in need of counsel, guidance, a leg-up.

There is no entrepreneur who is too big to have a mentor. A classic example is Mark Zuckerberg reaching out to Steve Jobs. The founder of Facebook was facing a phase of uncertainty in the early period of launching Facebook, and in fact, he had buyers wanting to take it over. At that stage, it was Jobs who advised Mark on focusing on his mission for FB and suggested going to India to seek his answers. Which he did. We recall a phrase that originated in the nineteenth-century in the US, 'Go West, Young Man', which urged people to go and look for fresh pioneering opportunities in the American West. In comparison, it seems ironical that Steve Jobs should advise Zuckerberg to go East—specifically India—so that he could reconnect with the mission of the company, a trip that Jobs had earlier undertaken when Apple was evolving.

Newspaper reports have described Jobs and Zuckerberg walking together in Palo Alto. Beyond mutual admiration, Jobs commended Zuckerberg for not selling out. Zuckerberg prized the advice from Jobs about developing a management team that 'focused on building as high-quality and good things as you are.' After Jobs' passing, Zuckerberg posted a simple tribute on his Facebook page: 'Steve, thank you for being a mentor and a friend. Thanks for showing that what you build can change the world.'

Zuckerberg once spoke about three key lessons in mentorship—sharing the mentee's enthusiasm for learning something new, investing even a small amount of time to open up a new world for someone else, and mutual gains through reciprocity. These lessons could be gleaned from an article published by the *Chronicle of Evidence-Based Mentoring*.

That mentors, in fact, could play multifarious roles was

the contention of Michael Sonnenfeldt, the CEO of a social networking site. He elaborated on this in his book *Think Bigger: And 39 Other Winning Strategies from Successful Entrepreneurs*. He categorized mentors as: the older, wiser veteran who shares hard-earned experience, the willing teacher, an educator eager to guide those on the startup path, followed by the generous peer who shares skill sets magnanimously with co-workers, and lastly, the soft-skills professional who offers structured mentorship.

Is some of this pro bono? Do we sometimes take the guru for granted? Is mentorship an act of generosity by big-hearted seniors eager to guide juniors? To explore these questions, we structured a session with a senior leader of a professional services firm.

He took us back to the classic scenario when trade and professions always had an apprenticeship model. The idea was that the apprentice would pick up the tricks of the trade in the hope that he would don the mantle in the longer term. However, he argued that with today's increased volume and complexity, and dismantling of geographical barriers, the traditional apprentice model is no longer feasible. With the nature of engagements being far more complex today, requiring multiple competencies, multi-competency teams are needed to solve specific client problems. A professional may be on one team today and a different team on another occasion. The individual professional, therefore, loses his or her 'stickiness' with a single supervisor. This could lead to a feeling of being lost in a large organization. It could also lead to a lack of mentorship to help or guide the professional in his or her professional development.

The solution? Assigning a mentor to each professional.

The mentor undergoes formal mentorship training and is responsible for the mentee's development. The mentee does not report to the mentor. The mentor obtains feedback from the different team leaders that the mentee has worked with. The mentor also understands the mentee's aspirations, provides guidance, and represents the mentee before the performance evaluation panels.

The ultimate aim: to groom the mentee into a future leader. But can the mentor let go?

At this juncture, I am reminded of a well-known Tagore song—'*Jodi tor daak shuney keu naa aashey, tobey ekla cholo re*'—which Rabindranath himself translated as saying, 'If there is no one responding to your call, then go on all alone.' Originally a Swadeshi movement protest song, it still resonates today. However, in the context of mentorship, I would slightly differ with its message—I believe a guiding hand is always necessary in both professional growth and life's journey.

The most telling examples are billionaires Bill Gates and Richard Branson, who sought out mentors. The Microsoft creator got Warren Buffet not only as his mentor but also as a philanthropic partner, something that Buffet stood for. When Branson was struggling to give wings to the fledgling Virgin Atlantic, he got Sir Freddie Laker, a British airline entrepreneur, as his mentor. It was Laker's mentoring and wisdom—especially in encouraging Branson to become the face of his company—that proved to be a game changer for the airline.

Talking about the importance of mentoring, Branson once quoted American entrepreneur Zig Ziglar: 'A lot of people have gone further than they thought they could go because someone else thought they could.' His takeaway from this?

Go out and find the right mentor to help you along the road to success.

Even someone like Oprah Winfrey, who's considered to be a self-made woman charting her own path to become a leading philanthropist and entrepreneur, acknowledges the importance of having a mentor. Summing it up in an interview in 2002, she said: 'A mentor is someone who allows you to know that no matter how dark the night, in the morning joy will come.' Oprah's mentor was poet and social activist Maya Angelou.

In our Indian context, we continue to abide by the established and accepted *guru–shishya parampara*—a long-established tradition deeply embedded in our various performing arts like music and dance, where the maestro and the mentee share a symbiotic relationship. Gurus, with the richness of their experiences and well-honed talents, are almost deified by their students, who practise art for endless hours, endure reprimands, and enjoy rewards, until they too become mentors in their own right.

There are several shades of difference between what constitutes an intern and a disciple. An intern is a young person who is in search of experience in an organization, often there to either learn something new or get a stipend or just for a resume boost, and is sometimes even absorbed in that company. With a disciple, there is a one-on-one disciplined interaction, where a teacher passes on his skill and lifelong experiences to a willing and talented disciple.

If we were to trace it to its roots, then the word 'disciple' itself originates from 'discere', which means 'to learn'.

From real life to reel life, countless movies have been made to highlight the plight and the passions of a learner, either in the corporate world, or in the creative arts space.

For this book, we have picked only two that demonstrate the variations in the approach to the mentor–mentee idea from different parts of the world.

The Intern, a sweet, sentimental movie depicting a reversal of roles, shows how a retired widower, played by Robert de Niro, becomes a senior intern at the ripe age of 70 in a company and mentors his boss, the young founder-owner of an online fashion business, played by Anne Hathaway. In contrast, *The Disciple* depicts the arduous journey of an aspiring classical vocalist (Aditya Modak) and his struggle for recognition and acceptance, guided by his guru (Arun Dravid) who preaches patience.

When it comes to communication techniques, the indirect mentoring also shapes professionals. Influencers and the beau ideals afford aspiring writers the impetus to improve their nuances, uplift their ideas, and make their manuscripts more ready for publication. Then there are mentorship programmes, structured writing courses, and master classes that give a leg-up to the aspiring writers.

A leading chartered accountant who is on the board of several companies talked about how, when he started, his boss would constantly criticize him—a kind of kick-you-to-improve mentoring which worked wonders.

I have a dedicated section, later in the book, where one can learn more from his wisdom, for this part focuses on the gurus who have shared their knowledge with those who have sought it.

13

Language: The Ramparts of Art

The artistic oeuvre takes on a huge sweep of forms
A lot of it defying the most established norms
It's no longer just a pretty picture
That gives life its tincture
But a language and lifestyle that weathers new storms

Art 'speaks' to us in myriad forms. The whole vast sweep of the word cannot be contained in a single canvas of expression. Broadly speaking, though, we are talking of art as produced over centuries—by legendary painters and sculptors—viewed at art galleries, pored over in richly illustrated tomes, acquired by collectors, discussed discerningly by art experts. Something that exists in an emotive mindspace.

But what about today's art scenario? There appears to be no limitation or inhibition in its presentation: inventive approaches, multi-dimensional art, public space installations, seamless transition into the virtual world, and with no travel restrictions, offline exhibitions thrive. Art auctions continue apace too and one continues to receive elaborately produced catalogues that are digested as much for creative information as for acquisitive pursuits.

Art certainly seems to cock a snook at the pandemic. Connoisseurs cannot be contained and artists refuse to hold back on creating. Commerce may have taken a hit but it hasn't been significant.

And there is no gainsaying the fact that creative artwork continues to make a splash, grab eyeballs, serving as a connecting force in a world that is temporarily cloistered.

In July 2021, the people of Rome were treated to a striking sight of an 18-metre cardboard bridge suspended by three large white helium balloons floating above the river Tiber. The Farnese Bridge, an installation by French artist Olivier Grossetete timed to celebrate Bastille Day, was made as a sign of Franco-Italian friendship. Its inspiration? A historic commission given to Michelangelo to create a bridge that would connect the Palazzo Farnese (now the French Embassy) to Italy. The cardboard was duly recycled.

However, there is much more to installation art or intellectualized art than temporary gimmickry. With this book, we will like to prise open the new forms of connective art space, emphasizing presentability, the importance of staying ahead of the curve, and reaching out to audiences for growing their minds—not only to expand their acquisitions but also to deepen their understanding of the art world through engagement.

This brings us to a space ideated over a decade ago in 2009 in the city of Kolkata, which has now become a strong metaphor for a new set of art movements that defy time, space and quantification. Experimenter, helmed by the creative duo Prateek and Priyanka Raja, wasn't what you would imagine a gallery to be in its traditional sense—flat canvases on walls waiting to be intellectually construed, acquired and written about.

Experimenter challenges those boundaries of visual art. Raja talks about its creation as: '...a space for free-flowing creative thought that challenged and provoked the viewers to think beyond the apparent, to question what they were made to believe and to reflect on contemporary moments in which we live. This is made possible with the work of some of the most inspirational and path-breaking visual arts practitioners from all over the world.' It is a place where difficult and uncomfortable questions are posed that have a huge contemporaneity.

While they do showcase paintings and sculptures, their scope is far broader. Embracing mediums today's artists work with, there is also video, performance art, installation, photography and other forms of artistic interventions. Their global programme brings together artists from across the world, unrestricted by geography or location.

Having been brought up on an old-fashioned, traditional diet of paintings displayed on walls and classical sculptures, one wonders if such art and artistry are commercially viable. And what kind of buyers come to appreciate this new dispensation?

Defending his turf, Raja says, 'An extremely well-informed and progressive audience exists out there.' 'Such practices find really wonderful homes in places that befit them. These are collectors who feel challenged by what they see, enjoying the exploratory avenues of thought that the works open up for them,' he adds. Many of these works find their way into some of the most prestigious contemporary art museums, as well as private and corporate collections.

Essentially, Experimenter acts as a conduit between its artists and museums and institutions—filling in the gaps in global art narratives and histories that have earlier been overlooked. So, this results in the communication being extensive and research-based, yet simple and precise. 'But what we speak is always rooted in knowledge. Art is a knowledge-based industry and if we are able to build knowledge leadership, we are able to communicate more effectively.'

Also, through their participation in art fairs—from New Delhi to Hong Kong and Dubai, as well as Paris, Basel, London and New York—the Experimenter brings audiences in contact with artists whose works they would not have had the chance to encounter and experience otherwise. Incidentally, Experimenter features impressively at 65 in the Art Review Power 100, the annual ranking of the most influential people in art.

Over the years, I have attended their annual Curators' Hub, a unique concept which delves into curatorial practices, the thinking and conceptual frameworks of exhibition-making, and perspectives of some of the leading curatorial minds in the world. The most defining feature of this Curators' Hub—which has become a part of the global arts calendar—is 'the breaking of learning structures as we know them, and a fearless and deeply intellectual space for dialogue and debate that it fosters.'

Their artist collaborations are unique too. Artists don't simply approach them, nor do they actively seek out artists in a conventional manner. Instead, they describe their artist relationships as akin to a courtship. First is the stage of the mutual attraction where they are already drawn to the artist's practice, followed by a period of exploration through group exhibitions and other projects. This eventually solidifies into a partnership. The process spans months and thousands of miles, but in the end the focus remains on the artist's vision, and the impact on the audience is the proof of the pudding.

The gallery is in fact 'fuelled through a fertile seedbed

of imagination and fearlessness that ignites with colliding yet potent possibilities. The bedrock of Experimenter is in its programming.' And when they celebrated their decade-long journey in 2019, the event reflected the deep relationships they had cultivated over the years—with artists, curators, musicians, media personalities, and the entire ecosystem coming together from across India and beyond.

Such galleries encourage debate, discussion and interpretation to bring in new perspectives. 'We never try to influence that perspective since that kernel is the artists' voice and we let it grow from there.'

As this book took shape during unprecedented times, we also explored how gallerists, auction houses, and international art fairs navigated that period with regard to their collaborations and commercials.

Experimenter, with their unique art space, felt it necessary to reach out to audiences in ways that transcended geographic limitations and challenged conventional templates. This led to the launch of Experimenter Labs, a laboratory-like space where research and experiments could be performed and new frontiers tested, as an 'incubator for future thinking'. Through the Generator Cooperative Art Production Fund, they extended fifty-seven production grants to artists all over the world to help them complete their projects through uncertain times. Additionally, their Experimenter Radio, which is a dedicated Spotify channel curating playlists, composed of music and podcasts by artists, writers, thinkers, curators, collaborators and philosophers around the world, brought an ever-growing offering of a mix of sonic experiences that act as sources of inspiration and reflection. The gallery has now expanded to a third space in Mumbai's Colaba area.

From Experimenter in India, we now move our focus to a neighbouring country, Bangladesh, which has witnessed some remarkable developments in the world of art. Interestingly, there's a link between the Rajas of Experimenter and the Samdanis of the Samdani Art Foundation, whose stories intersect at many levels.

Nadia and Rajeeb Samdani have also been featured in Art Review Power 100 list as amongst the most influential Asian figures in the contemporary art world.

In fact, they have been on the list since 2015, a recognition made possible because of the incredible contributions of all the participants of the last five editions of Dhaka Art Summit. This platform, founded by the couple, is something that I have witnessed evolve over the years. Artworks created for the Dhaka Art Summit (DAS) often go on to enter museums and biennale exhibitions all over the world, becoming a defining moment for many emerging artists' careers—both Bangladeshi and international. It is a platform which has captured the attention of the global art world.

The Dhaka Art Summit has become a crowning initiative in the region, showcasing the best of Bangladeshi art, while also inviting artists from neighbouring countries and bringing in top curators, auctioneers and gallerists to Dhaka to share their expertise.

The Samdanis have attempted to make art accessible to the common man while also nurturing artists by giving them a chance on a global platform. In 2023, DAS welcomed 672,000 visitors over a nine-day period. Later, one of its exhibitions travelled to the Kiran Nadar Museum of Art, India's first private museum of modern and contemporary Indian art.

The Samdanis recount how when they started collecting art together, they would visit different art fairs, exhibitions and biennales around the world. However, they found that there was hardly any presence of Bangladeshi artists. To the art world, South Asia was largely synonymous with India and Pakistan. 'Rather than taking Bangladesh around the world, we decided to bring the world to Bangladesh. Through the Dhaka Art Summit, many Bangladeshi artists have made their way to the international art scene—from important biennales and exhibitions to major museum collections.'

Nadia Samdani talks about how she would like to make Bangladesh the art capital of the world. Certainly, as a member of Tate Museum's South Asia acquisitions committee and its international council, and as the first South Asian (along with her husband) to receive the Montblanc de la Culture Arts Patronage Award, she has made significant strides on the global stage. In 2022, she was appointed as Member of the Order of the British Empire (MBE) and received the Chevalier de l'Ordre des Arts et des Lettres (Knight of the Order of the Arts and Letters) from France for her contribution to arts.

The couple have lent many works to various international exhibitions around the world and a few of Rashid Chowdhury's tapestry works are now part of the permanent collection of the Tate in the UK and the Met in the US.

Their personal collection is a story of its own. 'Golpo', which means 'story' in Bengali, is a magnificent six-level edifice which serves as both their home and a hub of their collection. Here, one can view art from all over the world in paintings, sculptures, installations and more. They initially began collecting for their home, but now they collect for spaces yet to be built and works that only exist as ideas. Much of their collection is for Srihatta-Samdani Art Centre and Sculpture Park—their future permanent art space in Sylhet, a region known for its tea plantations. Spread over 100 acres, this is their ancestral place, which will have multiple exhibition pavilions and a residency complex, committed to reach both local and international audiences. The initiative aims to invite curators, artists and writers from around the world to participate in exhibitions and interventions, as well as organize community-based activities. Best of all, access will be for the public.

The Samdani collection is eclectic, revealing cross-cultural influences of artists across South Asia and the world. Much of their collection is from Rembrandt etchings to Bangladeshi and Indian contemporary art. For instance, Ayesha Sultana is a Bangladeshi artist whose work they supported from the beginning (as did Prateek and Priyanka Raja of Experimenter). They bought some of her work showcased in Brisbane at the Asia Pacific Triennial—marking the first time this prestigious event included artists from Bangladesh.

During the pandemic, the Samdanis launched an online programme called *Art Around the Table* featuring weekly video workshops for the general public and children, contributed by Bangladeshi and international artists. Additionally, these online visits supported young Bangladeshi artists with modest fees, who then got an opportunity to showcase their work to international curators and collectors.

But one of their most fascinating initiatives was 'Concert from Bangladesh'. This was a multi-disciplinary and transnational digital collaboration to honour the fifty-year legacy of 'The Concert for Bangladesh'—the benefit concert organized by George Harrison and Ravi Shankar in 1971. For this concert, acclaimed British-South Asian artist Shezad Dawood created a virtual-reality stage which was streamed online and was followed by live events in the UK, the US, and Bangladesh. The performances were interspersed with archival and contemporary documentary footage, and the concert was amplified by augmented reality assets, including a free filter activated through audiences' phones and laptops, bringing 3D objects from their screens into immediate surroundings.

So, this is the new age of digital and augmented reality in art! And there's more.

Back in 2021, when the auction house Christie's broke new ground by auctioning a massive digital collage titled *Everydays: The First 5000 Days* by Mike Winkelmann, better known as the quirky digital artist Beeple, it went for a staggering $69 million: a historic milestone in digital art. How was it paid for? Ah! There lies the digi-rub! For us traditionalists, transactions in art now require one to be familiar with a new kind of currency—NFTs or Non-Fungible Tokens. For those who have been following and dealing in bitcoins, which are 'fungible', there are also NFTs or non-fungible tokens and these are connected with the use of this technology to sell digital art.

According to Wikipedia, a non-fungible token is a unit of data stored on a digital ledger, called a blockchain, which certifies a digital asset to be unique and therefore not interchangeable. NFTs can represent various digital assets like photos, videos, audio, and other types of digital files. Digital art was an early use case for NFTs because of the ability of blockchain technology to assure the unique signature and ownership of NFTs.

Yet, despite the rise of digital art, the three traditional Cs of Continuity, Collective action, and Creative extensions remain constant and timeless. The art world continues to thrive, both online and physically all over the world. Museums are opening up again, exhibitions and art fairs are getting new traction, and auctions, both online and offline, are robust. Art collecting, collaborations and experiential advances have not seen a halt in ardour and attention, nor suffered any attrition in patronage. Innovation is ceaseless.

And for connoisseurs of 'real' art, the skyrocketing prices at auctions are a tangible 'perfect presence'. For instance, in 2023, Amrita Sher-Gil's *The Story Teller* (1937) fetched a whopping ₹61.8 crore at an auction in Mumbai, becoming the most expensive work of Indian art on a world stage at the time. The women in the painting are intensely communicative. In 2025, an M.F. Husain work sold for over ₹111.8 crore ($13 million) at Christie's in New York, shattering the auction record for modern Indian art.

14

Laughage: Humour That Leavens Work Ethic

The comedian's a deep thinker, though he tickles funny bone
With jokes like javelin throws that land to dethrone
Your ennui and set rules
With humorous kilojoules
That can colour your world to relieve monotone

There has to be shock value, but also learning. Comedy is not a laugh-a-minute affair anymore. It is serious business and occupies a unique space that goes beyond tickling our funny bones to training and stimulating people's grey cells into focusing on the graver issues of life. It's a feather-touch approach to something that ultimately becomes a sledgehammer for getting people out of their complacent cocoons and into fresh perspective. Ultimately, humour is the yeast that makes life a lighter cake to digest, especially in today's worldwide scenario of gloom.

We focused on two people from the comedy canto, both celebrated in their specific applications of humour, both labelled stand-up comedians, but each inhabiting a specific area of engagement. One is Chirag Jain, known more popularly as Papa C.J., who is an executive coach and published author, and the other Anuvab Pal, who is a screenwriter, playwright and novelist.

Having known both of them since their growing-up years, there is definitely a sense of wonder at how they have notched up their successes in areas that our generation could not have imagined.

'No, you can't be serious,' is how we reacted when Papa C.J. announced that he was making a career as a stand-up comedian. Today, he says, 'When you're in love you don't really think. You just push ahead. And that's exactly what happened with comedy and me. I fell in love with stand-up and did whatever was required to keep the affair going. Ten years into the profession, I wrote a show called *Naked* during which I took off my clothes on stage and people paid to watch. So make what you want of what stand-up comedy did with my love for her!'

In his book by the same name, which has taken people deeper into their comfort zones (C.J.'s claim), it can be gone through in one sitting with the author's personal experiences serving as the draw. 'When they read about how I have been able to find joy on the other side of the challenges I have faced, it brings them catharsis and hope.'

And hope also comes through his commendable *Happiness Project*, through which he performs for terminally-ill patients in their hospital rooms. His life's mission is to uplift others and help them be the best version of themselves.

So, while the shock value of *Naked* has stunned us, there appears to be a take-home value too. How has he reached audiences during the pandemic times? C.J.'s answer is candid: 'I've always said that stand-up comedy is like sex—best enjoyed live and not watching it on screen. However much to my own surprise, over the course of the pandemic, I've quite enjoyed being a comedy "porn star".' Outrage, we guess, is the way to capture a person's immediate interest.

He has performed online for audiences ranging from 25 people to 7,000 families. The value addition, he feels, especially when the competition is essentially Netflix, comes from making the show interactive and the content deeply customized around the attending audience. 'As far as the take-home value is concerned, there is tons of science in place that validates the physical, mental and physiological benefits of laughter. However, I'd say, at a time when people are dealing with challenges, the likes of which they have never faced before, comedy and laughter help them de-stress and forget about their worries for a while. It also helps them carry that lightness of being with them much after the show is over.'

On the subject of using humour to make his clients think out of the box, he feels his experience and expertise exist 'at the intersection of creativity, communication, humour, business, leadership development and human interaction.' Working as an executive coach, he brings strategies from the world of performing arts to the table. In a *Harvard Business Review* article, he talks about how communication techniques that comedians use while performing can be used for pitching, fundraising and closing deals.

As far as humour is concerned, 'by its very nature, every single joke involves an element of surprise.' Additionally, it brings 'an intellectual perspective, empathy and humanity—all of which are a vital part of responding to the unexpected and adapting to new realities. Humour helps with communication, making an impression, navigating difficult moments, persuading others, shifting mindsets, unlocking creativity, acknowledging mistakes, building trust and being authentic. So whether you want to charm or disarm, humour is your friend at home and in the workplace.'

Can the grimmest of situations be defused with the infusion of comedy? For him, any subject is fair game for comedy, but there must be some empathy and sensitivity practised. His thumb rule is never to make another person's identity the prop, plot or punchline. 'You should always punch up, i.e. never pick on anyone or any group perceived to be weaker or the minority. Also, the general formula is that comedy equals tragedy plus distance, where distance includes time, geography and psychological factors or personal experience. So, you may not want to do a joke about 9/11 if it is immediately after the event (time), in New York (geography), or if you are aware of people in the audience who were personally affected by the tragedy.'

Coming back to the corporate scenario, we wanted him to describe a typical set of situations where he has been able to motivate a corporate group into upping their ambitions and vision. One example he gave was of a learning and development head who approached him to be interviewed as part of a learning event. He was taking on a new role in a new region and thought it would be a nice session to have early in his tenure. By the end of the conversation, he had in place a long-term plan with a series of interactions designed to showcase his organization, boss, customers and himself in a highly favourable light.

In the corporate training sessions, each participant has in hand a piece of paper with a tailor-made strategy that they can immediately apply to their current situation. Executive coaching, on the other hand, involves one-on-one interactions that take place every two weeks, with the engagements lasting for a minimum of six months. So, these are more customized and goal-oriented.

With an MBA from Oxford University, he wears many hats, including marketer, ideator, communications specialist, and brand and content strategist for companies. What does this entail? He runs, for instance, a show called *A Comedian's Guide to Communication Strategy*, where he maps out marketing and content strategies for corporates. He's also helped CEOs with their speeches. They come to him expecting humour, but what he offers instead as a value add-on is more around structure, storytelling and making sure their speech or presentation 'lands' and has the desired impact.

As an executive coach, he has worked with over fifty blue-chip companies globally and across cultures in over twenty-five countries, and has been invited to speak at Harvard Business School. With awards for Asia's and India's best stand-up comedian and performances with over 2,000 shows on stages that include full houses on Broadway and at the Sydney Opera House, the stuff of humour should be on an upward graph in both corporate circles and for a public in need of life's lighter moments.

Anuvab Pal's entry into the comedic space started out very differently. And perhaps this is a lesson for those who view straitjacketed careers as rigid paths, to break out of their blinkered thinking and consider the fluidity of change. There was Anuvab Pal, an investment banker who then went on to a career with Reuters and, finally, with family business issues coursing through his veins, returned to focus on the home front—specifically getting involved in the running of India's only floating hotel, the Manor Floatel. The hotel was designed to combine the best qualities of a luxury cruise ship with the beauty of a world-class hotel, permanently anchored in the heart of Kolkata.

But then, at 35, he needed to take the plunge, not into the waters of the Hooghly on which the Floatel stood uniquely, but into a creative space that was bottled up inside him.

'There's a lot you can do in the corporate world but a lot of it is indirect and in collaboration with other people. I felt I was ok but I didn't excel at it. Scriptwriting and comedy have a certain challenge—you are directly connecting with an audience. And being judged. It is like being in a circus. And I love the thrill of that.'

As a corporate stand-up comedian who has performed 400 shows, mostly for Fortune 500 companies, what could be the takeaway value of these shows? Was it something that went beyond entertainment to problem solving?

Pal believes that he noticed in many of his corporate shows how people often feared communicating with the public, especially when it came to public speaking. Pal talks about the fact that people laugh at something that has a kernel of truth. So, when he joked about something in the corporate world, people laughed but also introspected.

'Sometimes, it needs an outsider to introduce radical ideas in an industry because people within it either don't notice or are too busy. One of my favourite memories is doing a whole bunch of shows for the Tatas and seeing how they always laughed at the ridiculousness of the very English etiquette that the corporate world has. I guess because they were a company with a lot of proper etiquette. However, no one internally could point that out. They were okay with me saying it because I was an outsider—a comedian.'

Cut to Pal's expertise as a playwright, novelist and screenwriter. He sees these as entirely different worlds. We questioned him about two of his works which were highly commended. '*Loins of Punjab* is a comedy about a bunch of people taking part in a singing contest in Edison, New Jersey. *The President is Coming* is a movie about seven young Indians competing to shake hands with President Bush on his visit to India. However, both are just character studies. I am interested in characters and follies and my influence in film comes from the English theatre and Calcutta and all that.' With comedy, he likens it to being a musician—live and direct—where telling jokes feels like singing songs, where you play your greatest hits.

Apart from these, he has authored a number of books like *Chaos Theory*, *FATWA*, *1-888-Dial India* and *Disco Dancer: A Comedy in Five Acts*. The last is a spoof on the cult dance drama that was a hit with audiences over three decades back.

One of his hugely successful series has seen Anuvab Pal taking on the British Empire, which started as his one-man act *Empire*, presented in Soho and later at the Edinburgh Fringe Festival. He also did two episodes with comedian Andy Zaltzman on a radio show called *Empire-ical Evidence*, which traced the Crown's legacy through its physical remains in London and Kolkata. The radio comedy he wrote, titled *The Empire,* premiered on BBC Radio 2, with an eclectic voice cast, including Michelle Gomez from *Doctor Who*, Rasika Dugal—whom Indian audiences know from *Mirzapur*—and actor Stephen Fry.

The one aspect that concerns us the most now is connectivity, especially in pandemic times. All their shows have had to move to Zoom. 'Not only did the humour have to be interactive, but it also had to "feel" like a live show, bringing humour straight into people's homes. There were so many technological things that we did not have to learn because we could simply gather in an auditorium. Now, we had to adapt—whether it was learning software, lighting or even framing for a computer camera. Suddenly, everyone's home had become a digital studio!'

Even with scripts, where web series have taken over film, Pal attempted a play and a web series shot entirely on Zoom—the latter streaming on Amazon. The shooting, editing, casting of actors for the full eight episodes was done without even meeting the people face to face.

In fact, for artists like Pal, they travelled to whichever country was open for business, and he feels that artists and sportspeople were among those who were hit the hardest, having to juggle entry requirements for different countries.

But the most important thing about the reach of comedy is its ability to introduce new ideas and alternate thinking about a subject that can be applied to people's day-to-day work—whether in banking, coding, relationship management, HR, law, amongst other subjects. Pal's insights are eye-openers for today's mindsets.

'If you look at where corporates are turning to today for learning, they are no longer looking at some boring MBA professor. They are looking towards thought leaders like Warren Buffet or Elon Musk or even Bollywood stars. Their social media is followed religiously. There is a new term born out of social media called "influencers". These people, sometimes not even older than 25, include comedians, fashion lifestyle commentators, stock market gurus, and self-help and mental health podcasters; they are the new philosophers, thinkers, guiding the new generation of employees/audiences. It is all on the phone now. Gone is the era of endless engineering or MBA classrooms, chartered accountancy exams or IAS exams, as the way forward in life. Today, it is all about self-employed entrepreneurship. And corporates want to learn from them so that they can make their organizations more tech-friendly and innovative.'

At the end of the day, we would say, **never judge comedians by the number of laughs they generate, but by the disruptive spaces that they have created**—to give food for thought and action to their corporate clients, educational institutions and general audiences, tempered with the enjoyment and entertainment factor. It is a comedic cerebration that stimulates the mind which exists in a niche space for cogitation.

15

Linkage: Engaging through Music

The performer always impresses on stage
And his music becomes a huge rage
It's when he reaches beyond
To create wider bond
With the hopefuls that makes him true sage

Music can resonate with everyone, but when it also becomes a means of connecting and communicating with a larger community, that is when it can go beyond tuneful to purposeful.

When the pebble of the idea for this chapter about communication as an agent of change did a glissando across the waters one was testing, the ever-widening circles became symbolic of the keys of change. This idea lies at the heart of a musician of extraordinary calibre, Panos Karan.

Introducing himself on his official website, Karan says: 'I studied music for six years at the Royal Academy of Music, and while I learnt so many things about the music I am playing, the most fundamental question of "Why do we play music?" was never answered. In my twenties, after performing three solo recitals at Carnegie Hall in New York City, and in search of answers, I packed an electric keyboard and a generator in a canoe and sailed down the Amazon River of Ecuador and Peru, in order to meet new audiences and connect with them through the music that I deeply loved. This was the beginning of Keys of Change.'

And so he began on a journey to discover what music could truly do to bring about change. Setting out on a musical expedition, he didn't seek concert halls, but explored the most challenging corners on the planet, like Sierra Leone, Siberia, Uganda, Nepal and northeastern Japan. India was also a special part of the agenda. 'It was in Tohoku, Japan, playing for the survivors of the 2011 disaster, that I experienced the tremendous hope and encouragement music can give in times of the deepest crisis. Responding to requests of young middle-school students in Fukushima to come together for a performance, in 2012, I created the Fukushima Youth Sinfonietta.'

So, is Panos Karan a philanthrope or a pianist or both? It is entirely possible to combine the two as a musical ensemble, much like an appassionato sonata. I first met this classical pianist, who is also a conductor and a humanitarian, when he was on stage at the Calcutta School of Music in a concert a decade or so ago, playing with a fellow Greek flautist, Zach Tarpagos. The audience was enchanted, not only with the quality of the music they played, but with their elegance and the eloquent manner in which Karan spoke. His Greek god-like looks added to the swoon factor. And we applauded the presentability quotient.

The duo agreed to an informal interview, from which I could glean an entirely different side of their musicianship. Shedding their formal attire, I witnessed them taking to the streets to work with students from deprived backgrounds.

They performed without the glam but with compassion, in numerous places that included slum communities, schools for children of sex workers, orphanages, music schools, hospitals, homes for the elderly, etc. The aim was to reach out and play for them, and use music as a tool of communication and positive interaction.

In fact, on subsequent trips, they worked with classical musicians of Kolkata who came from less privileged families, but who actively played Western classical music as part of various orchestras in the city. Karan got in several musicians from overseas and had them practise with these local musicians. And finally, a grand concert took place at one of the important auditoriums in the city.

Karan's ideas are fast changing the understanding of classical music in the twenty-first century. Originally from Greece, Karan currently resides in London. He has visited more than 130 countries, speaks seven languages, and has also lived in Barcelona, Buenos Aires, Athens, Tokyo. While he has performed at some of the top concert halls around the world, his real impact lies in the places he has taken his music to—from the prisons of war-torn Sierra Leone to the evacuation centres of post-tsunami Japan. One of the most haunting images we carry is of him in a boat, with a giant keyboard, braving the waters of the Amazon and reaching out to people who need it the most.

In this book, I explore the multi-dimensional aspects of communication, hence it only felt logical to reconnect with Karan to understand the psyche behind going beyond making music, to helping and enthusing communities to rise above their wretched conditions. He imagines a sunnier world where music is brought to people, helping them connect with one another, and where it lifts them into a self-belief. A world where music can be created, whenever and wherever possible.

This is reinforced by the musician himself: 'Putting on our nice tails and white bow tie to please an audience that buys an expensive ticket is one thing, and it is an important thing indeed, as it is in these conditions—in the best concert halls in the world—that our music has reached the levels that it has. However, it is not the only purpose. Music can flourish in the rainforest, it can touch hearts in a slum community, and it can change lives in a children's home. It can do that and more, just like that, without the bow tie, without the pomp and circumstance, without the expensive ticket. I have seen it many times, and this, in short, has become the reason for playing music for me.'

In fact, when I connected with him in the beginning of 2021, he was doing a series titled *Bach Around the World*, where the videos and links show him play selections from German composer and musician Johann Sebastian Bach's work in various countries while introducing their history, cultural background, food and environment. It was the best way to get out of lives at a standstill and connect with some of the things that he loves most—music and travel.

I recall one instance which I particularly liked—actually all of them are standalone concertos where travel and music meld.

I tuned into part 11 of his musical journey around the world, where he can be seen at his piano playing a soulful *Bach Prelude and Fugue No. 11* in F major. 'Join me,' he says, 'as I travel to a place of infinite natural beauty and exotic mystique, in order to explore underwater treasures and ancient cities, and indulge in desert safaris, where the centuries-old Bedouin tradition meets modern finesse and luxury. This is

Jordan.' Spliced with quiet humour, there is even an image of him reading a newspaper as he floats in the salt-packed Dead Sea.

When I asked him to give other instances of these specific locations, he shared an anecdote about his musical visit to Ghana. '*Leave No One Behind* resonated with me as I moved my conducting stick up and down in front of a group of young musicians in Ghana. My music score was covered in dust, my hands sweaty, and my body tired from the heat, but I was proud listening to the sounds of Vivaldi, Beethoven and Strauss this youth orchestra was creating. They had been trying hard to improve every day, to work closely together, and to present a performance of which they could be proud. Living in a home, two hours away from Accra, that provides care for vulnerable children that cannot stay with their families—in many cases victims of abuse and other very grave circumstances—these children had been told too many times what they cannot do, what they will not achieve, what they are not worth. This time, together with three more music teachers all from three different continents (Australia, the UK and Mexico), we were there to show these children what they CAN do.'

So, did their work in Ghana have a deeper impact, apart from presenting a high-level musical performance?

'This project was an invitation for young people of very different backgrounds to come together and learn from each other. Most important, this was a call for young people to feel empowered and develop their leadership and collaboration skills in the process.

'For the musicians from the home, most of whom have endured trauma, it was a much-needed opportunity to connect with others, to feel safe and the sense of hope for tomorrow.

We saw how the trust within the group evolved as the days unfolded, how personalities softened, how interaction improved. We saw how the more experienced musicians started helping the beginners, and how the care for the whole group replaced, at times, the constant demand for individual attention.

'Perhaps out of proportion, but while I was working with these young musicians, I couldn't help remember how many times I was told by music teachers what I will never do. In this orchestra, everyone was welcome, and if they tried hard enough, they could do anything: complete beginners shyly joined, and in a matter of days, they were able to play a symphonic repertoire. Cliché? No. Anything is possible.'

We now turn to 2021, and the scenario shifts to Fukushima.

'The years have passed, and this January brought more than half of the students in the orchestra joining for the first time. Most of them are very young. They do remember the earthquake, but they remember the aftermath and the years that followed even more. Perhaps their family lost their livelihood as they couldn't sell any products from Fukushima anymore. Or perhaps they had to relocate, and find themselves in a new school where someone from the "hot" zone near the accident could be bullied. Or perhaps, after ten years, they are still living in a temporary accommodation provided by the government. Once the door of the rehearsal room closes, however, we are all the same: musicians, getting ready for a concert.

'As is the tradition with this orchestra, we chose some very difficult pieces of music and began working. Many of the new players had been learning their instrument for only a few months, but that didn't stop them. What seemed impossible at first became more than possible within a few days. "They never give up," says my friend and colleague Masanori, who is in Fukushima with me to help with the rehearsals and concert. The musicians of the Fukushima Youth Sinfonietta have been part of a musical revolution. While the rest of the world might have thought of Fukushima as a nuclear wasteland, young people from the region came together to share with the world that they are alive, active and creative. Their message is clear: Music brings them together; music helps them move forward. Music makes them better human beings.'

Despite the pandemic, Panos Karan collaborated with musicians in Chennai. Working with a local partner called Musee Musicals, the project is titled Chennai Youth Sinfonietta. It is a first-of-its-kind youth orchestra and will showcase talent of international quality.

All this is a far cry from elegant formal performances in famous halls around the world. Showing that it is possible to get your palms scuffed in the process of hand-holding of the less fortunate, but who can be injected with the promise of making music, adding to their life learnings, while igniting aspirations.

In a distressful world, such islands of musical equanimity might just be the balm for frazzled psyches, with music uplifting moods. And in knowing that through initiatives like Keys of Change, there is still an effort to reach out to the disempowered.

16

Montage: Photogenic Travel Primping Empathetic Perception

A picture today is worth ten million likes
When it comes from the traveller who gears up and hikes
The communicative vein
Will be never in vain
When there's changing perceptions through shared story strikes

Life is a prism. People view and perceive its facets through their individual perspectives and ever-changing perceptions. When we decided to see how communication could be upscaled in photography, music, art or film, it was a chance to find people who had gone beyond the ordinary to create new spaces, enhanced perspicacity.

And so, we go into these forms of communication with people who have been there, done that, but are now doing a sharp focus on augmenting perceptions through their chosen areas of passion.

'Don't blink or you will miss something spectacular,' is what Kounteya Sinha emulsifies in his philosophy. He has been a traveller all his life, as a 'journalist, photographer, storyteller, and as an ardent student of the world.' Sinha was *The Times of India*'s award-winning UK and Europe correspondent, with over 14,000 articles and 16 million hits for his posts. Most of all, he has been photographing with a mission, and a visionary eye that captures much more than what the immediate scene reveals.

But this is not about being a photographer as such. 'You have to also understand that we live in an era of social media. The phenomenon of what I call the "common man's photographs", everyone taking photographs, really hit the roof once the smartphones came in.'

In this scenario came one of the most innovative ideas that went beyond an individual photographer's mind space to become more inclusive of people around him and get them to experience something where the founders and avid travellers, Oiendrila Ray Kapur, Gagan Kapur and Kounteya Sinha, posed searching questions: 'Where have you been? Where are you now? Where do you want to be? Do you know what really matters to you? What do you remember of your life? What are your significant memories? Are they of the things you own or the experiences you have had?' Hence KOI, Bengali for 'where', happened—a child born during lockdown. It emerged from a need to escape.

'KOI intends to create a basket of experiences for a person that collectively creates an everlasting memory,' explains Sinha. 'We are nothing without our memories. The act of living far outweighing the act of the struggle of daily life. KOI uses food, places, people, towns, colours, walls, rainbows, roads and bends to create a memory that will make a person's life worthwhile. KOI is about being free from everything that holds you back from making a memory.'

On every trip, guests are accompanied by a group of highly trained and respected photographers who document their journey non-stop. I have personally seen a lot of the pictures posted by friends who have gone on some of these trips to places from Kashmir to the Andamans, Kabini to Chikmagalur and Bandipur. They are of National Geographic quality. Many of them have told me that what they like best is the entire photo shoot coming for free as a gift in a pen drive, superbly edited, when they travelled with KOI. It is all a part of my belief in bonding and connectivity, and in the impulses of this small band of individuals who have created a platform for people to experience and expand their discernment of the mundane from the marvellous.

'The primary DNA of KOI is based on the scientific evidence of visual memory and its importance. We know from various scientific studies that 65 per cent of people globally are visual learners. Our brain reacts and understands an image in as little as 13 milliseconds. We are capable of remembering 2,000 pictures with at least 90 per cent accuracy at any given time.'

Thus, they don't just take people to places but treat them to an overall experience and the act of making amazing memories. 'When they look back at the travel, they don't remember a monument or a landscape but everything that came about while visiting that place—the song they heard, the food they ate, the stories they shared, the people they travelled with, the friends they made.' With children who go on these journeys, the educative that goes beyond textbook learning is humungous. So is it for adults, especially those who may not have travelled in this adventurous way before. 'Most people think of travel as a holiday. It is freedom and escape, the act of breathing beautifully, the act of living to the hilt, the act of being experiences-rich rather than materialistically affluent. It's liberation as much as it is exaltation.'

Social media, then, becomes an important platform when people post pictures of themselves from a stunning location. Suddenly 'their rather lukewarm relationship with social media and their followers becomes a raging riot.' It brings in a different high. And when these guests travel to amazingly offbeat locations with KOI, dine in forests rather than restaurants or swim in turquoise blue rivers rather than under showers, they inspire others to embrace the outside world with open arms.

Kounteya Sinha's Project Bismillah is something that has resonated with a huge audience because of his rediscovery of the true essence and heart of Kashmir and the people's psyche. Here we reproduce in toto what Sinha has experienced, shared, grieved over, and brought to light through vibrant photography, which has had an effect on people who have joined in subsequent KOI discoveries.

'Images and photographs are repository of memories. Trips end but memories stay in the form of images. My experience with how photographs change perception truly came before KOI was born. It was with this incredible idea called Project Bismillah which I started. It was on Kashmir.'

In an interview with *Outlook* in 2024, Sinha said: 'Kashmir is an intrinsic part of our anatomy, ours to keep, ours to glorify, ours to savour and its fate, ours to keep. I have been deeply touched by Kashmir's scorching warmth, with its unparalleled hospitality and natural beauty, several times before. And hence, I was adamant that instead of sitting in our crimson carpeted drawing rooms, ruing Kashmir's fate that is mostly imposed on them, I shall, in fact, help change it by opening people's eyes.'

Project Bismillah was, therefore, 'the use of creative arts—photography to music, storytelling to films—to fight negative propaganda in a place of conflict.'

Project Bismillah was initially started by Sinha for love. Post August 2019, when India revoked Article 370, it became a responsibility. The internet was cut off, the military moved in, and Kashmir and its people disappeared from our lives— there was no contact with the outside world whatsoever. Tourism plummeted, the industry crashed, people lost their jobs, and for months, children and youngsters didn't go to school or college, had no television or phone, and no one earned a rupee. All of this was done for a better future.

But what about the Kashmir of today? What happens to the people today?

'The greatest tragedy of a place is when we forget them. Nothing destroys it like isolation. Abandonment, as a result of conflict and disaster, man-made or natural, causes its decay. This is when cultures, customs, tangible and intangible traditions, and folklore are lost. How long can a tearing performance last in an empty theatre? Bismillah by definition means "in God's name I begin",' Sinha told *Outlook*.

He heard so many people discuss Kashmir but how would those conversations really help people on the ground? That's when he decided that he was not willing to leave it alone. He became part of Project Bismillah.

'Project Bismillah is about photographing Kashmir— travelling to the far ends of the state—discovering villages and people off the map, ultimately culminating into a body of work that intends to remind the world what unimaginable beauty runs through the veins of Kashmir. And the strength of their comebacks,' he says.

'Post Article 370 abrogation, saffron production in the valley, which accounts for 90 per cent of the total yield across the country, suffered. Terrorists killed lorry drivers who went to Kashmir to bring apples—an industry that supports over three million people in the region. Fruits fell into drains and were destroyed. However, the tenacity of the people in Kashmir is made of sterner stuff. They had seen all of this before. They knew misery loves company and hence they didn't give a damn anymore.

'On the ground, children played. Families stocked up for a long winter. And in the midst of such hardship, when ration was measured, every home we passed by opened their doors and offered us food and drink. The warmth was more scorching than the summer sun.

'I had to do something for them. Project Bismillah was born at this moment. It was our way to give back. No threats existed, but people refused to go there. Propaganda said it was unsafe. It wasn't,' Sinha added.

As India's top art critic Uma Nair said: 'Project Bismillah has now become a rage. It is being talked about everywhere across the world. Papers are being written on it, on how the visual arts can truly play a powerful role in bringing a place of conflict back to its feet.'

When he started releasing all the images of Kashmir, people were inspired to travel with him and when they saw Project Bismillah and its visual imagery, they became Kashmir's ambassadors with earlier suspicions of safety deleted from their psyche.

That is the true power of images. Another aspect I have gleaned from talking to Sinha and his team is how people have started taking themselves seriously, at giving themselves a chance at glamour or at being able to be noticed.

So, when a group, mostly of women in the sixty-plus age group, went on what was dubbed as the Silsila trail, they emerged as divas in their chiffon sarees emulating Rekha in the 1981 film with the same name. There they were, traipsing through the tulip gardens, dancing and posing, with abandon showing on their faces and with gestures reiterating how wonderful it was to be alive, to be independent, to be ecstatic. The photography team believed in the philosophy of kindness. They were taught how their act of clicking a shutter would not just create a photograph, but could change the way a person felt about themselves.

Changing perceptions, making people believe in themselves and having the world come closer, are some of the things that Sinha's own philosophy has infused into the new travellers. As a 'documenter of the world, people, places, circumstances, emotions, regular mundane life to the exciting upheavals of society,' he has brought in a new sense of personal documentation.

During a visit to the Obeetee factory, renowned for its luxury carpet and textile brand in Uttar Pradesh's Mirzapur and owned by Rudra Chatterjee, Sinha traversed remote terrains to uncover the story of the region's women weavers. He then unveiled a rare repertoire of work called 'Fate Lines—How the Thread Changed the Destiny of Mirzapur's Women'. The show opened in the hallowed portals of India's most coveted gallery, the Bikaner House, and saw the who's who from the world of politics, diplomacy, governance, arts, culture and fashion land up mesmerized by what was on display.

From India's G20 Sherpa Amitabh Kant to Mahatma Gandhi's granddaughter Tara Gandhi, from the Ambassador of Rwanda to the Director General of the National Gallery of Modern Art, along with top designers like Tarun Tahiliani, Shantanu and Nikhil and J.J. Valaya—all left behind rave reviews.

According to a blog on Obeetee's official website: The show of 65 stunning photographs taken by Sinha unravelled sensational stories of women from the hinterland, who fought societal norms and patriarchal practices to come forward and work against all odds, changing the social fabric of the region. None of these women had stepped out of their homes till 2017. In a rare rebellion, to become the breadwinner of their families—with their husbands either alcoholics, gamblers or just unwilling to work—they decided to step out, learn the ancient art of carpet making, and have now become the torchbearers of a change in society.

Nearly 2,000 women have now become phenomenal weavers. Sinha discovered all these women and more importantly, for the first time ever, got them to open up about their lives from behind that veil.

Uma Nair in her column for *The Times of India* reviewed the show and said: 'It is an epoch-making journey that goes behind sumptuous carpet stories to unravel the beauty of feminine fervour. Kounteya Sinha has a rare gift—he can sniff out the spectacular from even the most mundane. Kounteya as an artist likes to slug it out—dig out stories till his bones ache. The photographs and stories of tremendous resilience and triumph of these women—many of whom have now become the sole bread earners of their family—are vignettes from everyday living. Unparalleled in his craft and brutally honest in his narrative, Kounteya spins stories that stand testimony to time. His penchant for the extraordinary, his intellectual prowess emerge from his extensive experience and nuanced understanding of the world, in an odyssey that covers over a hundred countries in search of stories, with the world as his oyster.'

In 2023, one of the events conducted on the sidelines of the G20 meet was curated by Sinha at the world's oldest tea garden—Makaibari in West Bengal's Kurseong. The tea estate is also owned by Rudra Chatterjee, the chairman of Obeetee. Sinha and his KOI director Oiendrila Ray Kapur created one of India's most iconic and largest murals—the 175-foot *The Wall of the People*, celebrating the invisible tea pluckers—leaving the delegates from twenty countries awestruck.

The mural, spanning the length and breadth of the factory façade, was created in a record time of less than a week. It is spectacular in its storytelling and is vibrant beyond measure, with portraits of real pluckers of Makaibari, first photographed and then recreated through art. The artwork also immerses viewers into a visual extravaganza of the region's flora and fauna, boasting of over a thousand species.

The year 2023 saw Sinha bag some of the world's most prestigious awards. He received the most coveted Nelson Mandela Leadership Award at St Hilda's College, University of Oxford, as Photojournalist and Visual Artist of the Year. He again won the Brand Guru of the Year at the India Excellence Awards, Delhi, and at the Pride India Awards, Bengaluru.

We present this chapter as an inspiration to reflect on past experiences through photographic evidence and move beyond pandemic times to enhance connectivity. `**With greater self-confidence acting as a catalyst for personal upliftment, we hope these stories encourage outreach and engagement, and help open doors of perception and set in motion the windmills of people's minds.**

17

Plumage: The Soft Feathers of Entrepreneurship

The globe is their oyster, where they show extra edge
With new ventures, and vision, and big bucks as the pledge
It's all theirs to mine
But their hearts are on shine
To go beyond profits and give philanthropic pledge

Hard hat, hard-nosed, hard-hearted. The first denotes not just the protective headgear worn in factories and construction sites, but also stands for entrenched conservative belief, almost melding into the second—with its uncompromising stand. And being hard-hearted, of course, shows callousness and a lack of sympathy.

Why do we lead with these negatives? Because there are also hard-hitting entrepreneurs and investors who are positively changing the face and pace of the startup ecosystem taking it to dizzying heights. And then they reveal their soft-centre, somewhat like the crispy outside jalebi oozing its sticky sweetness at first bite.

We're talking jalebi at this juncture quite contextually. Did a lot of people not groove to the music of 'Jalebi Baby', which amassed over 200 million global streams? This coincided with the path-breaking IPO of food aggregator Zomato.

It was surely sweet music to his ears, with the digital release of the 'Jalebi Baby' rap by Tesher and Derulo in a way heralding Zomato's ground-breaking IPO, as Info Edge founder Sanjeev Bikhchandani found his investment in Zomato leap up 1,050 times to ₹15,000 crore. Some telling facts: Shares of the food aggregator Zomato, which were issued at ₹76 in the initial public offer, closed 66 per cent higher at ₹126 apiece. Zomato's market capitalization on day 1 of listing rose to nearly ₹1 lakh crore. And Info Edge now holds 15.23 per cent stake in Zomato after selling 2.32 per cent stake through the Offer For Sale (OFS). Meanwhile, the music video featuring Zomato's cameo (we will come to that shortly) had over twenty million views in a week on YouTube.

Apart from these dizzying stats, to us this was a real triumph of communication—gaining popularity and acceptability for a product that has been a winner in the food delivery sector. The jalebi, too, got a renewed traction—'looking like a snack, looking like a whole meal'—borrowing from the words of the rap song to repopularize it internationally. We are left wondering why there is no geographical indication for this vastly popular sweet—twisted to an art, syruped to death and perked up in the craziest shades of tangerine. A national favourite, it holds centre stage at wedding reception live counters, is as much an early morning staple as it is a snack for all times and seasons, and should definitely be boosted over the 'hot cakes' phrase.

The series of events that unfolded saw Zomato getting featured in the worldwide release of the *Jalebi Baby* music video by Canadian-Punjabi rapper Tesher, which was later remixed for wider global appeal by American singer-songwriter Jason Derulo. With millions of views already, we won't be giving anything away by mentioning the storyline which shows Tesher and Derulo as restaurant waiters trying to woo a pretty customer who has placed an order of jalebis. Tesher, clumsy with his jalebis, drops them on the floor, when Zomato comes to the rescue with Jalebis in a brightly-branded box. They rush with the order, only to find that their beautiful target has eyes for another! With lavish sets, brocade sherwanis and extravagant costumes, the video is a visual treat, where Zomato emerges as a true star.

But the real hero of the story is Deepinder Goel and his team. We will come to that story shortly. First, let's talk about Sanjeev Bikhchandani's journey, and how his uncanny intuition worked right from the beginning and shaped India's leading digital ventures. Anyone who has ever searched for a job, looked for a matrimonial match, explored educational opportunities, or scouted property, has come across or turned to one of his hugely popular websites. These platforms—Naukri.com for jobs, Jeevansaathi.com for matrimonial alliances, Shiksha.com for education, and 99acres.com for property—are all part of India's most trusted tech enterprise and the first Indian internet company to be listed on domestic stock exchanges, Bikhchandani's Info Edge.

The person behind all this is the founder and chairman of Info Edge, Sanjeev Bikhchandani—an investor, creator and mentor, and now a philanthropist, with his investment in Ashoka University, one of India's top liberal arts institutions. With a larger-than-life personality, a no-nonsense attitude and infectious optimism, his ventures reflect his 'win-you-must' attitude.

His investment in Zomato is a tale worth retelling. Especially considering how Zomato's Deepinder Goyal and investor Bikhchandani are now amongst India's super-rich after the food aggregator's spectacular IPO.

More than a decade ago, Bikhchandani's Info Edge had invested ₹4.7 crore in Zomato. Back then, Deepinder Goyal was running a website called *FoodieBay* through which customers could find restaurants and order food. Bikchandani was one such user, but being the entrepreneur he is, was also seized with the idea of investing in the website. He went about it the hard way—he found Goyal's email ID through a Google search and sent him an email offering to invest in FoodieBay. Within three days, they struck a deal. Fast forward to the current times, Bikhchandani's investment has paid off a thousand-fold. A quote from the investor is a modest way of acknowledgement: 'The credit should go to the Zomato team. Our skill lies in merely identifying great teams and putting in money. Money is a commodity. Entrepreneurship is rare.'

Deepinder Goyal is now amongst the crème de la crème of the super-rich, with a personal fortune that is close to a billion-dollar mark, following the record-breaking success of his IPO—one of the largest in the startup sector to date. And the self-made Bikhchandani, a Padma Shri awardee, now commands a worth of more than $3 billion. Goyal was also on the judges' panel of the much-watched business reality show, *Shark Tank India 3*, which premiered in 2024.

As for Bikhchandani, we view him not just as an investor with a huge appetite but someone with a keen eye for detail—which is at the base of his success.

When Policybaazar came into his ken in 2008, his meeting with the founders was the trigger to shake hands on a deal he felt could be immensely workable and he went ahead and invested in it and saw it become a unicorn in a matter of ten years. In 2021, PB Fintech Ltd, the parent company of Policybazaar, an online insurance aggregator, opened its IPO and raised ₹5,625 crore ($700 million).

So, there is—to take the jalebi forward—a huge sweetness to the whole investment scenario. It got its biggest boost ever and should be seeing more capital flowing into the ecosystem. The encouragement to startups will surely have a ripple effect. As Bikhchandani tweeted: 'Here is the ultimate evidence why India should invest more behind its startups and in early stage VC funds.' He talks magnanimously about how he sees the floodgates opening for other startups to go for an IPO. It has shown, according to Bikhchandani, that a startup 'need not domicile and list overseas in order to succeed.'

Many of the lessons we learnt, as we talked to the likes of Bikhchandani, were their single-minded customer focus, the flamboyantly cautious risk-taking ability, and a nugget that readers must always carry with them in their search for perfect solutions—the meticulous attention to detail. Once when he was talking to the owner of Burger Singh, he delved into size, specification and other minutiae. On a broader educational canvas, when he invested in Ashoka University, he persuaded the board to 'stick to the knitting' and focus on making it a pure liberal arts college, rather than going into a multi-disciplinary institute.

Peer acknowledgement backs this up. He could be perceived to be ruthless in his interaction with startups. Instead, he has been accommodative, transparent and flexible. One of the Policybazaar founders talked of his 'ethical compasses pointing to the north'. And with Deep Kalra, the MakeMyTrip founder, his sense of corporate governance and ethics was hugely lauded, particularly when Bikhchandani was on the board of his company.

In fact, Kalra recalls how in the mid-2000s, his company MakeMyTrip had ramped up business in ticketing but had not grown in a related area of activity, the holiday packages market. Bikhchandani's advice was to get back offline by opening physical stores so that customers would find them a trustworthy option for a complete holiday package which would go beyond a mere sale of tickets. Some board members were uncomfortable with such suggestions, but it worked as a magic wand, getting them multiple national outlets and a deeper understanding of the Indian consumer.

In our emailed interaction with Kalra, we wanted to know what really propelled him to become an angel investor after having gone in for a lot of mergers and acquisitions. Had he reached the zenith of his achievements?

'To be an angel investor,' he replied, 'you have to be curious, a student for life, have an appetite for risk and ability to accept failure. As an entrepreneur, I want to play a part in spawning a new generation of entrepreneurs and I am happy to play a role in the evolution of these promising businesses. So, be it to provide a network of contacts, assist with recruitment, serve on the board of directors, and mentor or coach the management team, it's gratifying to be a part of the larger startup ecosystem.'

In the context of what we are trying to prove in my book, we asked what was the main thrust of their promotional interface with potential customers in the travel arena and USP vis-à-vis competition. Did they just serendipitously carve out a unique space?

He felt that MakeMyTrip's biggest differentiator was their

ability to address diverse travel needs and demands of the Indian traveller on a single platform, as a one-stop shop for all things travel. So, it was really about focus and specialization.

We came across a recent set of CSR activity from Kalra to improve the quality of life for the populace of Gurgaon, where he lives. Because it is these small acts of concern, by individuals who are running large businesses, that are the real gems of contribution to society.

'I fundamentally believe that the world we live in needs our attention and care, and every act of social good is important to help us make the change for better. Committing yourself to a cause you feel passionately about and starting somewhere is important—even if that means starting small. That's the philosophy and I hope the work done by MakeMyTrip Foundation inspires others to consider paving it forward.'

Today, with his two-decade-long journey as an entrepreneur, he has learnt 'immensely from successes and way more from failures.' 'I thoroughly enjoy contributing as a mentor, advisor and an angel investor, and will continue to work within the Indian startup ecosystem, finding more value and meaning by nurturing entrepreneurial dreams.'

Kalra, like Bikhchandani, is one of the founders of Ashoka University and is a part of its governing body. In fact, it was Ashish Dhawan, an Indian private equity investor and philanthropist, who founded Central Square Foundation, a grant-making organization and policy think tank focused on transforming the quality of school education in India, and who spearheaded India's first liberal arts university, Ashoka University, with the support of more than forty philanthropists—Bikhchandani, Kalra, Pramath Sinha of Harappa, amongst them.

The early years of setting up the university were detailed in a lengthy and highly memorable session for students—which we watched online—between Bikhchandani and Dhawan. They talked about how the focus from the beginning was for a liberal arts university, and not mixing it up with other disciplines. Dhawan mentioned how Bikhchandani has been adamant about it. 'Had we gone down the other path, liberal arts would have been the orphaned child.'

From quantitatively successful verticals to quality education—there is plenty to chew on.

We come back to the presentability factor, where Bikhchandani was clear that it should be on a firm foundation of substance. As for the perfection quotient in life, his philosophical take to us was: 'I don't think perfection is achieved. The ideal is what keeps it going. **In a changing world, perfection is a moving target.**'

18

Rampage: Of Startups Serenaded by Angel Harps

If its music to your ears, it must be angels up on high
Who are waiting at the ready for the startup guy to fly
Ideas can't be lacking
So why not get cracking
And burst into action to make their dreams fructify

The startup scenario in India has never been better than it is today. When we think of a startup, it is no longer the straggler or the would-be entrepreneur with an armful of ideas but no clear direction. Starting up and scaling up, pitching it to an angel investor and getting accepted—there is so much that is aspirational both in the air and on the ground.

So, gone is the somewhat hopeful glint in the eye and in its place is a thriving scenario of startup companies that have enriched India's entrepreneurship ecosystem. These sentiments of positivity have come through in one's interactions with individuals who are in a prominent leadership space—the investors who are funding, growing, mentoring startups and even helping the aspiring entrepreneurs get beyond their bootstrapping blues.

One such individual stood out for us in the angel firmament. You could not miss the magnetic presence of

Padmaja Ruparel in a room. A few years ago, at a conference of The IndUS Entrepreneurs (TiE), a non-profit organization started in Silicon Valley, when a group of startups was making their pitch, much in the manner of the Shark Tank process, it was Ruparel who quite blew us away with her quick-witted reactions and on-the-spot decision-making; some of the young, green-behind-the-ears hopefuls actually secured higher funding than they could ever imagine.

What else could you expect of someone who is nationally recognized as a key player in the Indian entrepreneurial ecosystem, is the co-founder and president of the Indian Angel Network (IAN), and gained recognition as one of the Top 50 Most Powerful Women in Business by *Fortune India*? She has also been listed in *Forbes India*'s W-Power Trailblazers amongst other encomiums. Apart from being an active angel investor, her operating experience spans large corporates, mergers and acquisitions, and startups at their very early stages. She is co-chair on the board of Global Business Angel Network, and a seat on the high policymaking tables in government and on the SEBI working committee ensures enhanced national credibility.

I caught up with her over a lengthy interview when this book was taking shape and I was focusing on what angel funding was all about, to see where communication gaps existed. Ruparel said she got into angel investing well before anyone knew about angel investing in the country! 'It was by accident,' she said.

To elaborate further, Indian Angel Network (IAN) was a first of its kind for India and is acknowledged as one of the world's largest group of business angels, made up of a whole bunch of successful entrepreneurs and top-level chief executives from India and overseas.

Initially, the baby steps saw half-a-dozen members pooling in not more than ₹10 lakh to ₹15 lakh to invest in startups. This set the ball rolling for a greater number of investors coming to them and their investor group starting to grow bigger. 'As a country of 1.3 billion people, we think of scaling genetically. And we started considering how we can bring investors from around the globe to invest in entrepreneurs from around the world.'

And so, IAN was built in a manner that within a decade it soared to become a global institution. It now boasts nearly 500 investors from a dozen countries and a portfolio of over 180 companies in seven countries, across a wide spectrum of sectors, with operations in six cities, London included.

So, how does the IAN model work? It is a full-service model for investors which goes from the pipeline of investment opportunities to divestment. There is also the IAN fund, of which Ruparel is the founding partner. It is a uniquely differentiated ₹375 crore fund, which has created the largest horizontal platform in India for investing in seed/early-stage ventures, attracting high-quality entrepreneurs. Which sectors are the gainers? The fund, according to one report, 'invests in innovative companies in sectors including healthcare and medical devices, VR, AI, software as a service, marketplaces, fintech, big data, artificial intelligence, biotech, agritech, cyber security, etc. The fund leverages and builds upon the strengths and success of IAN, the world's largest angel investor group, to breed and grow innovative companies.'

There's no such thing as an overnight success in this particular arena. Ruparel's first investment was in the oil and gas sector and got 20 times returns. But she did not pay too much attention to it. At Xansa, an outsourcing and technology company, she led corporate communications and brand building strategy. It was at Xansa where she met her life mentor and guide in Saurabh Srivastava. He is a founder of the Indian IT industry, serial entrepreneur and investor. The company was acquired by an FTSE 100 British company listed on the London Stock Exchange. With this, new challenges emerged for the Indian company for brand building, as now the Indian company could not announce new clients, among other restrictions. She, therefore, came up with the idea of increasing visibility by creating softer stories focused on corporate social responsibility (CSR) which ensured the company was in the news every calendar day. In addition, the CSR programme became central to client engagement and retention strategy.

There could be a lesson in this for startups that have gone to a certain level and could stand apart from the crowd in their incorporation of CSR as part of their strategy.

Apart from volunteering with NASSCOM, India's software industry association, where she met many icons of the Indian IT industry and built relationships, which would help her later in life, she helped operationalize the Delhi chapter of TiE. This was a unique step for Ruparel, to connect to India's very nascent entrepreneurial ecosystem. It is here she met people like Kanwal Rekhi (legendary entrepreneur and investor from the Silicon Valley), Raman Roy (the father of Indian BPO industry) Sanjeev Bikhchandani (Info Edge founder), Deep Kalra (founder of MakeMyTrip), amongst many others. She also helped operationalize the Indian Venture Capital Association—India's first and now largest association of venture capital and private equity firms.

On the subject of how investors sense a 'good' product—is it intuition, or based on how smart and complete the plea package is? Should startup founders be less arrogant? Do they look for passion, vision, perseverance and an ability to deal with failures? Ruparel feels that it is important to empathetically understand the entrepreneur and gauge whether he is fully committed to his venture and confident of the space in which he or she is building the venture, and is yet open to new ideas and able to convince the investor. They need to be confident but not over-confident, and there is quite a bit of 'gauging the person' the investor needs to do.

Talking to Ruparel is like unlocking a box full of stories: we learnt that one entrepreneur's deal/term sheet was cancelled at the last minute when the investors found the entrepreneur was travelling business class whereas the investors were travelling economy. It got nixed probably because it pointed to lack of capital efficiency!

However, she feels it is also important for investors to frame questions in the right manner because if the investor declines, maybe he or she has not really got into the heart of the presentation. A big idea presented with panache could definitely win over a brilliant concept that is poorly communicated. One of the things that need to be factored in is when should the company go public with its product, or leverage media/social media? Ruparel believes it is best to go public, offline and online, only after the startup founder has some customers, and is able to deliver on this front. Once sorted out, they need all the PR and communication to help scale up.

When we wanted to know if an angel investor looks at the following Ps (as different from the normal marketing Ps)—pitching it right, preparation, perfection in credible presentation, and perception management, Ruparel felt the fifth

'P' was crucial—passion which could take the entrepreneur forward.

During lockdown, did she see a new resilience and what sort of businesses would qualify to get considered by angel investors?

Ruparel elaborates, 'The pandemic forced us to change and adapt for the long term. Virtual became real, with in-person meetings having become almost impossible with physical distancing. Hence, online socializing became imperative: video meets, LinkedIn, Twitter, Instagram, etc., becoming primary ways to connect/network!

'And therefore, it has become important to find a balance between the formal and casual, and between the serious and non-serious. It's critical that our communication, however brief, has the right words, tone, correct spellings and grammar, and balances ease and respect. Many of us in the startup world are in a hurry and take our online messaging lightly. However, it puts us on the back foot from the word go! For entrepreneurs, online/video pitches are here to stay and honestly, it's a huge advantage.

'These are time-efficient and have a wider reach for both investors and entrepreneurs.

'What will be the "door opener"? It is still the pitch deck—a sharp, clear, focused deck, which is well-researched. This must provide all the data on market size, competition info, delivery model, financials, team background, risk and risk-mitigation strategy, among other important details. Everything matters—the format, font, colours, and number of slides. This is what will bring the investor to dial in on the video call. At the investor pitch session, it simply doesn't make any sense to 'read' through your slides. If you find it difficult to talk to blank screens, as many people don't switch on their video, get your co-founder to switch on theirs!

'As the investor starts to get a handle on your business plan and you are interrupted with questions, welcome them! This is the best endorsement of investor interest. While it is important to answer the questions, it is also imperative to admit when you don't know the answer—it is your chance to demonstrate integrity.

'While you may have prepared the perfect closing remarks, adapt quickly: ensure you have addressed all the questions and responded to the queries/clarifications asked as promised. All of us are at home and we dress casually, but when you are presenting, it is important to project a sense of purpose and seriousness. It doesn't mean you need to wear a suit and tie, but a dishevelled look won't really help your cause either. Your body language matters, even on a video.

'You also need to ensure what is visible on your screen apart from yourself—you don't want an open toilet door to be in the frame!

'It's very useful to pre-check your laptop, video link and connect with the organisers a day ahead of the meeting—and again fifteen minutes before your pitch. Technology engages but when it malfunctions, it disengages very quickly! It is important to research your investor: understand which companies they have invested in and highlight the value-add you would hope for from the investor. That's a key engagement point and will usually secure you the next meeting!'

At the end of the day, it is more exciting than ever to be an entrepreneur, with new opportunities emerging all the time. It is also a hedge against the loss of corporate jobs. The gloom and doom are now behind us, replaced by a new adventurous streak to step up in the startup space. And of course, what we set out to prove from our PR point of view—**the need for structured communication, a positive mindset and a presentability quotient—to nudge out the competitor or win the confidence of the investor.**

19

Rivage: Transparent, Continuous, Cohesive Communication

There can be no full stops when you communicate
Verbalizing, connecting should ever be in spate
Immediate and true
Open-minded in hue
For switch-offs can only cause trust to abate

Many of our crisis communication manuals could bite the dust unless they adapt to the many new challenges that the pandemic threw up for communicating with multiple stakeholders in a fast, furious, but fraternal manner. During the pandemic, the spotlight was on political leadership to minimize fear and increase faith in the system, on the medical professionals to share blame and soothe a panicked public, and CEOs who carried the can for employee connectivity in a warlike preparedness. This is where we set out to find how this urgent sense of connection between CEOs and their employees unfolded in the corporate world. So, I reached out to someone whom I have observed over time for his approaches and accessibility in keeping his workforce motivated.

When this book is published, we will be well away

from the fears and the terror that was generated during the pandemic. The interview was conducted at the peak of the crisis and we record it for posterity.

Harshavardhan Neotia is the charismatic chairman of the Ambuja Neotia group, one of the most prominent and respected corporate houses headquartered in Kolkata with a diversified business portfolio in realty, hospitality and healthcare. The author has seen his unique approach of engaging with people for a good three decades, and the pandemic was the time to find out how the worst crisis of our times was tackled by this corporate leader.

So, on to some pandemic prescriptive. Harshvardhan Neotia's motivational communication started out with a letter to employees, and then went into the video format, which were open, transparent and inspiring. How was he able to convey both the downside as well as engage in the doling out of advice to keep up confidence levels?

Neotia was candid: 'The Covid pandemic caught the world by surprise, spreading like wildfire and causing fatal illness and economic hardship for individuals and organizations alike. The virus tested everyone's resilience.

'This may sound motivational rhetoric, but I have always believed that "it's not what happens to you, but how you react, that matters." During these trying times, not once did I think or feel that it was over. Of course, I was concerned and so were my colleagues about their future. I did what I could to alleviate those concerns. I shared my plan and openly discussed what we were going to do. I told them it would be hard work but promised that if they were willing to go along with the plan, we could ride this out together. I also said we would be back to normal one day, but it wouldn't be soon. My best guess then was 2021. My new best guess is now 2022. Six months from now I may change that again. I'm optimistic, but I'm also realistic.

'I realized everyone needed to have confidence in their future, otherwise they would be paralysed with fear. I do check on my team members and have made one-on-one a regular part of my routine. I tried to give them a sense of confidence and realistic optimism, following which they were energized and our relationship strengthened.'

He mentioned that he tried to be more visible than ever before. To this end, he said, 'I filmed more short clips, arranged more "ask-me-anything" type of Q&A opportunities, made sure more company-wide emails than usual come from the top to keep people informed of business bright spots, and so on. These signalled to my employees that everything is being done, as best as we can, to mitigate the impact of the pandemic.'

Since we are concerned with the regularity of methodology used in communicative tools, like the magazines and newsletters that are produced, we needed to know if these really have assured continuity and a sense of connection amongst executives.

Neotia is emphatic that communication is key to any business. 'Without a healthy dialogue between departments, between stakeholders, customers, government officials, investors, manufacturers and clients, organizations would find it difficult.'

'Magazines and newsletters are an important component of effective marketing and branding. We share these magazines with our employees and contacts because it creates a friendly collaborative atmosphere and work culture, enhances bonding as well as gives comfort to our clients. Embedded with helpful links, a catchy heading, captivating designs as well as visual descriptions, they convey group information, the progress and developments across different verticals in a simple and concise manner. They also reflect the group's sensitivity towards culture, art, and community as well as positioning of brand "Ambuja Neotia" which aims to make a difference in the way people live by being sensitive towards people, planet and processes.'

When companies grow large, how do owners and CEOs ensure getting employees on a common platform? Is there an annual day which, perhaps, gives a chance for employees to exhibit their creativity? While this may not have an immediate bearing on our discussions on communicating during extraordinary times like the Covid-infused situation, yet it is important to know how normal situations also keep a set of corporate executives motivated.

Neotia has always encouraged bonding through team-building exercises and outings. He feels that the Ambuja Parivar Annual Day has been a good way to interact with employees and their families, but that it has not been possible of late for obvious reasons. However, apart from the annual day event, he says, 'we also have town hall get-togethers where I personally share the developments as well as challenges while interacting with the employees. We also used to have an annual offsite conference where HODs across business verticals spent two days sharing their progress, learnings and future plan for the year.'

'As an organization, we value sharing our learnings and the initiatives being taken to harness that through multiple interactions. These events help me get to know my teammates better, and find out what they want—both of which I use to identify ways to motivate them. I have tried to create a friendly, collaborative work environment by showing appreciation and recognition for a team's (or an individual's) hard work through simple thank-you notes, tangible awards, and celebrations.'

Neotia says, 'Organizations work best and are most satisfied when the team is working together, very tightly, with the same understanding of what exactly they're trying to accomplish. If everyone shares the same vision of where they're heading, why and how, then it's much more likely they will adapt well to the changes and challenges they're inevitably going to face.'

But coming back to the pandemic, there is one area where many corporates have jumped in with philanthropic intent to add to any measures that could alleviate health and other related issues. A compassionate communing, to be able to make a realistic contribution.

'In the pandemic, we all saw examples of people looking out for one another and doing whatever they could to ease others' troubles. Businesses pivoted to provide lunches to children who were attending virtual school, acted with agility to accommodate customers' unique needs, and threw their weight (and financial support) behind social movements. We, too, felt something needs to be done to support the city's healthcare ecosystem and give back to the community.'

And so, the company converted a small piece of vacant land in New Town into an oxygen-enabled 58-bed Covid care facility christened Vinod Neotia Covid Care Centre. Obviously, it worked better through a tie-up with local organizations and NGOs to ensure a smoother reach. And here's the beauty of it—patients coming through their reference did not have to pay any bed charges.

The company also offered thirty luxury bungalows of their Ffort Raichak resort to the state government to be used as a quarantine or isolation or medical facility. They did not think of the commercial aspects and extended their facility to strengthen the state's preparedness in coping with the rising demand for medical infrastructure in the first wave.

'As an employer, I did all that I could within my means including arranging for free vaccination for all employees, special medical leave, support for next of kin, and providing accommodation facility for self-isolation (in case of non-availability of rooms at their residences). We also helped employees who needed medical support not related to Covid.'

This narrative is not complete without showing another facet of Harshavardhan Neotia—the cultural connect, which, we found, has a bearing on the persona of someone who has a leadership status in society. Workplace connectivity is one thing, but there should also be a cohesive communication in other areas, as the title of our chapter suggests. In Neotia, we found that there is also the person who helms inspirational musical videos, giving his voice to it, delivers speeches in multiple languages, and participates in everything from theatrical productions to heavyset web-based discussions, and publishes volumes of creative literature annually on areas of cultural import. Are these all part of a larger macro picture of communication through different paths?

'I was born into a family which is deeply interested in fine art, music, literature and philosophy. As a child, I participated in conversations and activities associated with music, art and literature. Even today, I love to be part of cultural events hosted by my friends and business associates.

'Considering my growing-up years where each member of my family has been an art aficionado, design comes naturally to me. I am a proponent of arts in all its forms, I have tried to reflect this in the edifices I build. We try to incorporate art in many projects, especially hospitality ones. I am also a staunch supporter of most things local. It reflects in our landscaping also. We attempt to ensure that the surroundings continue to thrive much after we have dusted our hands off the project.'

But coming back to the stressful times that we are faced with, Neotia feels that the 'tumultuous nature of the past year—if not longer—has given credence to the idea that change is the only constant. Although the business world has been feeling the pressure to build more diverse and inclusive work environments over the past couple of decades, the pandemic and social unrest in 2020 magnified the importance of these efforts. Business leaders like me were backed into corners and forced to take tough decisions about priorities and trade-offs, general welfare and profits.'

So will the nature of business and industry and the world of commerce face a sea change?

'The business landscape will only get more complicated in the coming years with increasingly disruptive technology and events. No matter the industry, companies will face unexpected changes in the future that will require quick thinking and creative problem-solving—just like some of the issues faced during the pandemic, including the mass exodus to remote work and creating digital and contactless processes.

'We, too, looked for a way to leverage our expertise, diversify our service offering, protect our revenue stream and better serve our clients. We are growing and adding new clients every month, but it hasn't been easy. It has taken effort and humility. We learn new lessons nearly every day. One of the biggest lessons is to not become complacent. Keep evolving. Try new things. Fail fast and move on. Despite all odds, we try to delight the customer by crafting aesthetically designed spaces for a memorable experience.'

It is perhaps these aesthetics that form the core of Neotia's sensibilities that is reflected in his projects as well as the decor of his own home and office spaces, thus creating a kind of gold standard for others to emulate. In fact, his intuitive and imaginative work in social housing earned him the Padma Shri.

'Real estate projects, for me, have never been about creating an icon, but about making a built structure that is in harmony with its location and surroundings. It also meant marrying social and environmental responsibility to aesthetic ambition.

'I am extremely passionate about design and architecture. It is a subject close to my heart. I try to use unique and aesthetically appealing architecture and design to add value, to complement the lifestyle of buyers, and for better urbanism.'

We reel back to the importance of open communication and the leader's willingness to share wisdom. Are heads of companies sparing more thought on the immediacy of communication?

'I am sure all company heads are doing it in their own way and style. Improving employee engagement is crucial for creating a diverse environment of flexibility and community building. I spend more time with my work family than my real family, and to ensure that my companies are successful, I encourage trust, communication and understanding, just like I do at home. I hope these help in better performance, better employee retention and better productivity.

'When life-changing things happen outside the workplace, especially during working hours, it's hard to tell employees—be it the company's president or a porter—to handle their emotions outside their workday. I encourage my employees to talk about their feelings, concerns or conflicts in a judgement-free zone where they can rely on the support of their co-workers and managers.'

And he continues to communicate on a national level in his leadership of industry bodies. Because leaders like Neotia epitomize substance, style and sustainability, our book sets out to exemplify such traits in individuals for readers to be inspired into getting to the acme of achievement.

Neotia reacts by talking about the numerous things: 'We will have to leave behind as we embrace the new normal after the pandemic, but there are plenty of lessons we need to carry with us. These lessons alone will help us lead an agile, innovative company that embraces the unknown.

'Covid notwithstanding, we have always focused on creating projects that are sustainable, from the way they look at the site and systems, to design materials that are used in the projects. Sustainability and green initiatives have always taken centre stage in all our projects. Going forward, I would like to remain true to our core belief—do things differently, maintain quality, take care of design aesthetics, and deliver what was promised.'

So, on one hand, it is a continuance of ethical, artistic work that is in keeping with corporate vision, and the immediate as well as long-term stepping on the gas to motivate a large set of employees and stakeholders through our critical times, on the other, that could win the day. **Hope is that hard-hat that workers keep on, and faith is what leaders must kindle to keep the wheels of work culture alive and thriving.**

20

Sportspage: Transformational, Not Just Inspirational

You may change the person not his tone
And help them not to go alone
With coach as lead
Advice they'll heed
You guide, the rest is theirs to hone

In the charismatic world of sports, where you find a certain invincibility about players, there are as many instances of high performance as there are of failures, struggles, emotional issues, mental health. The transformation of mindsets and the rejigging of emotional upheavals through hands-on advice from experts in HR, on the field and off it too, are what constitute the new methodologies for survival and success.

We look up to and emulate sports personalities and ardently follow their games. But the shockers and setbacks that tumble out are equally distressing. When the 23-year-old Naomi Osaka, one of the bright lights in the tennis firmament, pulled out after her first round of success at the French Open at Roland Garros, there was awe all around. When she refused a media interaction post the match, citing stress-related depression, what kind of multiplier effect could this have on other high-performing players? This is a tennis star in her prime, a four times Grand Slam champion, someone who is on top of the endorsement charts, a *Vogue* cover girl, and, one would like to add, an opponent to be feared, deified too.

To clear doubts and get some cogent answers to the trigger behind such an act of withdrawal, I turned to Cape Town-based Paddy Upton, the 'Barefoot Coach' who, as the team's mental conditioning and strategic leadership coach, essayed India's 2011 World Cup win. In his new role, away from sport into advising on mental toughness and the personal well-being space, I asked Paddy Upton how he views such acts from Osaka.

When he works with an athlete, he says, the first thing he tells them is that he does not view them as an athlete, a superstar or even as someone special, as many of their fans might do. 'I see them as an ordinary human being, one who was lucky enough to have been born with talent for their sport. Talent is a gift from birth, so is not an accomplishment. The work they put into turning that talent into results on the highest stage is something they can view as an accomplishment and something to feel proud of. Still, this does not make them a special person, but an ordinary person with a special talent. They only become a "special person" when they conduct themselves according to values, ethics and character traits that would earn any "ordinary" person a high regard from respected peers. I explain this so the athlete can see that it is important to work on both at being a great athlete and on being a good person. Seeing themselves as an ordinary person also means that like you and I, they are also susceptible to naturally occurring insecurities, doubts, vulnerabilities, fears, etc.

'It is quite human to experience mental challenges under highly stressful situations, as happened with Osaka. If I were to work with her, the first thing I might do is to help her understand that it is normal and okay to experience what she is experiencing. I may help her deal with processing outsiders' views that hold the notion that it is somehow not normal for an athlete to struggle mentally. Next would be to work towards solutions, which are almost always available when one takes a smart and authentic approach to mental or emotional difficulties.'

Michael Phelps, the 23-time Olympic gold medallist, came forward with his support for Osaka, as he himself has had run-ins with depression and was empathetic about her vulnerability. He, in fact, went on to produce a documentary in 2020 focusing on athletes' mental wellness. Adding heft to this has been the sporting bodies being seized of the physical and mental well-being of athletes, illustrated by the International Olympic Committee's IOC Safe Sport Action Plan and the Mental Health in Elite Athletes Toolkit. In their toolkit, a large number of areas are covered—from anxiety-related behavioural disturbances, depression and sleep-related problems to alcohol misuse and eating disorders, to mention some. It was endorsed by none other than Olympic champion Abhinav Bindra.

In 2023, both Osaka and Phelps came forward during the US Open at an event on Mental Health and Sports. At the time, Osaka didn't mention when she wanted to return to tennis (after giving birth to a daughter in July). However, she did make a comeback in early 2024, following a fifteen-month break. Many other athletes have come out in the open about their problems.

How does Upton see these developments? He felt it was important for athletes to see themselves both as athletes with special talents and as normal human beings. So, there was the necessity of working to improve athletic prowess, whilst simultaneously embarking on a journey of personal mastery to be the best person or human being they can be. 'As their self-esteem grows, the more they become equipped to deal with two of the biggest mental obstacles to success in sport—pressure and fear.'

In his new advisory role for those seeking mental toughness and personal well-being, we got an insight into the resetting of mental mindsets. Individuals and those who are in work situations in the corporate world are under a lot of pressure to perform. And so, in taking a macro look at the pandemic scenario, Upton says: 'We do not know what the future holds, but this much we know—that we are all in the same boat. Since everyone is struggling to navigate in the current world, we are looking at what a person can do to be at the leading edge of the performance curve. And if you can get better upfront.

'One of the things common to the best athletes in the world is that they are their own best coach. They own the library of knowledge of their game, and at the same time, they are open to new learning from others, such as their coaches. This is a recipe for success. In contrast, too many athletes and employees rely on others to tell them what to do and how to do it. They defer to others to be experts in their lives, such as their coach or the HR department. This is more a recipe for mediocrity, as it leaves people handing over their power, decision-making and responsibility to others. And others can never truly know what is best for you.'

In the corporate world, people join one company and look up to one leader. But then the change of jobs, which is happening with metronomic regularity in today's world, alters the whole scenario. People have this tendency to hand over their homes to an interior designer or their bodies to a physician, without taking direct responsibility or relying on their own ability.

A vast majority of clients come to motivational experts like Upton when they need them the least. It lies in their hunger to grow. There are a lot of people who approach him when they are 'broken and need fixing'. But it is not the person who is in need who reaches out, but their parent or their boss who approaches Upton for advice.

I would like to rewind to the time of his life when his future ally in coaching, Gary Kirsten, was still in good form for his country. Meanwhile, Upton decided to go out of sport and move 'into business, philosophy, academia and spirituality'. That is when he pursued a master's degree in executive (business) coaching. He was exposed to a host of innovative companies, business leaders and academics in the world and started to gain a deeper knowledge of how to gain the best out of people. 'The best leadership philosophies employed by the best companies worldwide enable them to attract the best talent, keep them the longest, and simultaneously, to get the best out of the rest.' In today's scenario, the leadership approaches lean more towards people management and coaching, away from the old school command-and-control and instruction-based style.

I recall a session I had with Paddy Upton in Kolkata as part of my Red Sofa conversations which would have celebrities from all walks of life appear in a one-on-one conversation with me and the audience would be a handpicked one. We had based the session on a book titled *The Barefoot Coach* written by Upton which had its maiden release.

His coming to India in 2007, along with head coach Gary Kirsten, was a brief from the Board of Control for Cricket in India (BCCI) to alter the whole approach of the Indian team in preparation for the tournaments to come. The goal that Upton and Kirsten created for themselves was to make India the number one team in all formats of the game. Their success was unprecedented. We, as Indians, tend to be highly individualistic, and this is where they introduced a team culture, coaching the team rather than just the individual, 'where the environment could serve as the mental conditioner'.

There were many myths he busted for us at the time—one being the concept of mental strength. He said he had never come across a professional athlete 'who doesn't have fear, insecurities, vulnerabilities, doubts and negative thinking.' He added, 'But for some reason, there is this idea in the sports world that those things are bad and if you've got them, you are mentally weak, fragile and soft.' Not at all, that's normal.

There was never any let-up in the positive mindset of the coaches to goad the team on to believing they should win. They did everything in their power to prepare players for the time that was to come their way. At the session, he shared how he involved one of the greatest adventurers of our time, Mike Horn, who had conquered all parts of the world, even circumnavigating the Arctic Circle. Upton requested this extraordinary individual, who, at the time, was on his yacht somewhere in the Andamans, to come over to address the Indian team which was scheduled to play against South Africa in Kolkata. Horn interrupted his 100,000-kilometre expedition and rushed over. The insights and inspirations were to leave a deep impact on the team, who realized that having the will is one thing but knowing that you are capable of winning is a different ball game altogether.

So, are the new mantras all about transforming the negativity, changing mindsets, enhancing their innate talents?

Upton believes in an intuitive leadership, which is not an airy-fairy concept, not a go-where-the-wind-blows style of management. It means meticulous planning, but always being flexible to change direction.

Today, in South Africa, he is working a lot with parents, especially those who have high expectations and live vicariously through children. Children want acknowledgement, love and recognition from their parents, but not the pressure to perform. He is coaching parents to raise children with self-esteem and not focus on results.

This translates into the business environment. He focuses on getting people into a natural motivational flow. In business, you need a fertile environment. A leader has to keep removing weeds and the bad eggs from a corporate environment. You must have an understanding set of people and make sure they do not use yesterday's information. While accepting opportunities, the conditioning coach for corporates looks beyond toxic cultures, sifting through them, and accepting only socially responsible companies with whom he can work with integrity, credibility and passion.

'Harnessing the collective intelligence of a team is not just a strategic imperative for teams…it is also a path towards lasting contentment and better results in cricket, business and life.' A tactic that gels well with his new environment of business team building activity with the addition of wisdom and humility, 'getting off your high horse of all-knowingness and moving into the neighbourhood with your fellow men.'

It is heartening to see such humility in someone who has been a mental coach to professional athletes from ten countries and eleven different sports, an acclaimed speaker, a university professor, and is armed with degrees from four universities, including two master's degrees. Disarmingly self-deprecatory too. 'I am a wannabe surfer who loves fishing. I'm not as interested in cricket as I am in building, or attempting to build, extraordinary team cultures in high-performance environments.

'When an athlete approaches a season or career-defining moment, the understanding is that this is the time they need to bring their A game. Similarly Covid lockdowns and the associated economic, social, mental and physical health challenges have pressed almost every human being to bring their own unique A game to navigate these unprecedented times. The twist is that although the term "bring your A game" is commonplace, it turns out that nobody, not even Google, has defined what the core components are of an A game, in sport or life. I spent two months in lockdown investigating and interrogating the A game concept, and eventually, arrived at a six-part framework that is relevant to almost every adult, and can be used to guide people to find theirs. I am currently helping people in business and sport to build the content and story of their unique A game, using this six-part framework. The aim is to give each person the best chance of successfully navigating the stormy waters we're currently navigating as a global community.'

We have come over the uncertain times hump, so **the challenges are to continue growing core competencies, turn to professionals for advice and consent, and to keep the wheels of business and industry whirring**

with approaches that are conducive and do-able. While our example has been based largely on one transformational coach, and mostly sport-oriented, there are many management consultants and educators who are changing tack and track to be available to employees and students for counsel in the winning game.

21

Verbiage: Letter Literacy — the Write Way

The lettered are really the unlettered lot
Their messages are never the ones to be sought
The real-time mail
Is one that can't fail
If it's personal and regular and with emotion fraught

While we do not wish to take the extreme illiteracy route, the reason for dwelling on letter literacy is that we are at a strange crossroads today. Book readers are legion and authors continue to prolifically write, while publishing is in a constant state of reinvention. Online is overt. Lit fests have proliferated, self-publishing is the new art of personal trumping of the system, social media strategies give immediate short-term lift-ups to authors looking for a quick hype. Meanwhile, e-books, audiobooks, Kindle, etc., have their own touch, and poets and PhD-ians get their niche readership. The bestseller is the beast that never bites the dust.

But our cavil is against something that is fast disappearing. Simply put—it is the art of writing letters.

The short messaging service or SMS in its more visible form, which even the semi-literate can finger-tip execute, with its further banal abbreviations, has put paid to a once lettered communication scenario. There is also the stuff that gets sent on email, done in a hurry, without so much as a glance over for correctness, and often even dictated. CEOs largely delegate communication to an executive assistant, or a corporate PR person, and rarely does one take the trouble of writing a personal note—in appreciation, in condolence, or as an inspiration.

In defence of CEOs in our lockdown lives, now hopefully behind us, it has to be said that they have all been feeling the urge to reach out to their employees to assure them that 'Aal Izz Well'. I have come across some fine examples where the chairman or the chief executive has regularly sent out letters that inform employees about the difficult situation the company is going through, the need for belt-tightening, which owners are themselves undertaking, and alas, the temporary salary reductions they have resorted to. The letters then get into the mode of getting employees to address their stress-related situations and also encouraging them to use their work from home as an opportunity to pursue other talents. Some have gone to the extent of creating videos where the CEO was seen addressing executives—a warm and personal manner of coming before his people.

In all this, there lurks the hand of the corporate communicator, but to give credit where it is due, it has to come as a brain-spark from a CEO. He or she must surely initiate and instigate their PR communicators to execute, for they are meant to have the writing skills.

Over the years, in my corporate communication assignments with corporates, this has posed anguish and given confidence in equal measure. It has always been a tabula rasa—write that Directors' Report for the Annual Report, draft a chairman's speech, compose parallel communiqués to shareholders, employees and press for an impending merger, and incidental bits of patchy notes reworked sensibly. Input it all yourself. As wordsmiths, the enjoyment and opportunity lie in plucking inspiration from the air, or recalibrating what the lettered leader has a writer's block about. A lot of journalists have kudos and cash in the ghosting of autobiographies and books on institutions. That's a separate beautiful skill set.

But I go back to trying to create something out of nothing. The magic potion by Getafix that would make the Gauls feel like supermen. When the much-decorated and well-admired Field Marshal Sam Manekshaw was the chairman of the multinational company I worked for, and asked me to draft his speech, I was all agog, apprehensive no doubt, but ready to take on the challenge. When I took him the first draft, he looked indulgently at me and said, 'But dear, it does not sound like me at all.' It took several inclusions before the final product was shareholder-ready. Although he largely diverted at the press conference, that is another story.

Leaving those speeches and corporate necessities of communication aside, what we have set out to highlight in this chapter is the lessons to be gleaned from the men of letters who made letter writing a fine art. That, and also how any person reading this must become mindful of how they can personally address situations in daily life which requires them to put pen to paper, or through other electronic means.

So, when these letters were written and compiled and became de rigueur reading, what emerged was gleanings from history, the sharing of everyday and higher philosophies, and really, those that have become the stuff of high literary writing. In rewinding to our school days, there was something so pertinent, so personal, in Jawaharlal *Nehru's Letters from a Father to His Daughter*. It was a set of thirty letters written to his daughter Indira while he was in Allahabad and she was in Mussoorie. The topics covered were diverse, from going back to the formation of the earth to how human life came into existence, and the manifold faiths, beliefs, customs—giving a macro picture of human history, with a focus on Indian history. The language was simple and these historical facts were easy to digest. In later years, he also penned letters to the heads of the provincial governments in the book *Letters for a Nation: From Jawaharlal Nehru to His Chief Ministers*.

Conversely, in a college in the US one used to study the letters of William Faulkner to his mother and father, pretty much around the time that Nehru was writing his famous letters to his daughter. These letters were a storehouse of observations on the places he visited when he went beyond his native Mississippi to the further north of America and to Europe. The letters were later culled and crypted into the novels in his mature years, in the novels that got him high praise and earned him a Nobel Prize in Literature for his 'powerful and artistically unique contribution to the modern American novel'.

My personal letter-writing proclivities have a number of facets and face-offs to it. In the main, being an ardent believer in the power of a quick note, a long epistle, a pat-on-the-back message, or of course, the romantic rune, all of these have made their impact. But beyond the personal, I have actually formally introduced sessions in my training programmes on the variety of letters that can, and must, be written. One such session upped the interest in something that many young people had not ever really used—the postcard. I had purchased a bunch of them from a post office—the 5-inch-by-3-inch postcards. I pointed out how similar in size these were to their cell phones, which had become their undisputed companions for connectivity. The surprise on their faces was palpable. But the task that daunted them was when they were told to write to anyone they pleased, especially a grandparent, and actually go and post the letter. I got back one a week later, but with just a line saying: Hope this reaches you. Sigh! Could one lone piece of feedback ever be, perhaps, worth a half-a-day workshop?

However, over time, students and adult groups were impacted with the importance of sending thank-you notes to people whose homes they stayed in and availed of their hospitality, of condolence messages, handwritten letters to colleagues in appreciation, tailored covering letters for job applications, letters to gen-next in the family (I did an A to Z series for our son, when he went to college, to make it a little different, less preachy, but with roundabout exhortations slipped in). Conversely, my father, in his beautiful pearly script, wrote me this encouraging letter using an Osmiroid calligraphy pen as I was leaving for studies abroad. The letter is still part of my memorabilia, along with handwritten notes that some celebs—authors and politicians and academics in their day—sent with best intent.

The person who really excelled in calligraphic handwriting was Professor Purushottam Lal, a man of immense learning, the person whose knowledge and grasp and subsequently the transcreation of hundreds of volumes of the Mahabharata are precious additions to our understanding of the scriptures. Extraordinary was the fact that he was a one-man publishing house—having birthed the Writers Workshop, several decades ago, to publish new and fledgling authors, which resulted in thousands of volumes of poetry, prose, novels and translations that have given us a credible body of diverse work. Not just that, each book was hand typeset and covered in Bengal handloom sarees with the borders and motifs staying intact, and his masterful calligraphic handwriting was bestowed on the titles of the books, embossed in gold. Each book was a giftable proposition, apart from being meticulously proofread and containing massively readable contents.

Finally, allow me to speak of love. Love letters—not to tutor people into writing them, although the intent lurks. Not the mushy versions, nor the teary ones, but rather what became a series that seized the stage all over the world.

I first saw the Pulitzer Prize-nominated play 'Love Letters', written by American playwright A.R. Gurney, in the West End, and many years later, the Indian version in Kolkata, and one can only give it an eternity certificate. It has just two characters, in the American version, both born to wealth and position.

The format is unique which uses the 'epistolary' form, where the characters sit side by side at different tables and read out from notes and letters. Well-known actors and actresses have been known to take on these roles because it requires no committing to memory and are meant to be read out on the spot, on stage.

The Indian version, 'Tumhari Amrita', had a run for more than two decades. Its huge success was unprecedented in the realms of theatre. It toured venues all across India and the US, Europe, Pakistan, and the Middle East. The adaptation saw a fresh Indian context, done by Javed Siddiqui, a story of unrequited love read out through love letters between

Amrita Nigam and Zulfikar Haider, exchanged over 35 years, the central character of Amrita being based on bohemian Indian painter Amrita Sher-Gil. Its original cast with Shabana Azmi and Farooq Shaikh just blew away audiences for years on end, until the latter's passing. The play is so timeless and easy to stage, that it has seen performances on cruise ships and was staged in the UK during the Covid lockdown.

But the play apart, the whole point of the discussion is a love letter, which can, must and should be written at some stage, as long as roses and jasmines evoke perfumed fervour, as long as the pledging of emotive connect happens across divides. Romance is animate. Seize the day.

There is, then, a sense of timelessness to the whole art of letter writing that cannot be given short shrift even with the invasion of the 'Instagrammed' means of communication. There are many areas where letter writing persists, for instance when people write letters to editors. They find it a convenient platform to express their views, dissent and opinions on subjects covered in the newspaper, or issues of import. It is another matter that a handful of these letters get published, but that is part of the hazards of the fact that a choice has to be made from the thousands received on a daily basis. But the institution continues apace.

I have a friend, a self-professed Luddite, who, until before the lockdown, unfailingly sent picture postcards from wherever he travelled around the world, with a lot of details written in it. It was so personal, so pleasurable, and so different from the instantly clicked images and occasionally good travelogues that are publicly shared.

Lest I be accused of living in the past, there is no getting away from letters that can impact our lives. Letters of intent, going on to be translated into industrial licenses, letters of resignation (remember a play by this name that was based on the life of Harold Macmillan?) that can be penned without anger, but with emotion; letters of complaint—the well-drafted ones eliciting empathetic reaction and results.

In eighteenth- and nineteenth-century England, there existed letter writing manuals, which did not just instruct lovers what to say, but actually guided people about writing on business matters, as many of the people in that time may not have received the kind of education that would equip them to express themselves.

Here, we assume that **people have a certain level of understanding, self-expression, the desire for connectivity and commitment, the yearning to send out that missive, the need to write when things are going wrong, and the imperative to interface. That missive could be a change agent.**

If I have to use a pen, it is a simple Bic medium-point black, which suits my cursive well. But my real indulgence is to fill up my heirloom Mont Blanc with Quink and use a colour that reminds me of the waters off Mauritius—a turquoise blue that lifts up the senses.

It's the 'write' time to be letter-literate.

22

Voltage: Presentability over Mere Presence

She was a person of great learning—a sage
Her books with their wisdom were all a big rage
But at a prestigious TED Talk
Her careless couture made all balk
And she took a big hit on 'advantage image'

So, no matter what a brainiac you are, or are gifted in the various creative arts, the outward presence and presentability is as important as the knowledge or talent you are showcasing. In the many lockdowns, when a lot of people climbed on to Zoom and other bandwagons to express their views through group discussions, we noticed a significant change in appearance. People had taken the trouble to be well turned out, a mark of respect definitely to the rest of the participants. It also showed that individuals are seized of the fact that there is a certain credibility attached to a smart, studied presence that exudes a mental preparedness.

The proliferation of webinars was, in many ways, a boon for people to connect through a virtual platform. There is something dynamic about the interactivity that webinars afford. As the physical conferencing, once de rigueur for companies, took on the more compact and impactful shape of web meets, it became easier for individuals to jump into presentation mode with reduced preparation time—with the added incentive of appearing before audiences who would be actively tuned in. Apart from putting their points across more succinctly, those who were the lead players in the webinar had to be well turned out to wrest credibility and audience interest.

These sessions proved that the formal act of getting ready for a world outside the home need not be the timeworn method of preparing for 'official' appearances. Our mindsets were able to change to accept that good grooming begins at home.

In fact, this applies to women who are homemakers. They are multi-taskers, managers of kitchen, children, husbands and household planners. How do they look at all times? Haldi-stained saris and faded kaftans are no longer meant to be the trademark of a cookery queen. If queen she must be, attire should be fresh, with a face to match. The lady of the house is the leader of the pack. Looking fit and good, and acting positive are the signal for the rest to follow.

The innumerable cookery shows that hog viewer imagination have shown just this: the presence and the ability to demonstrate are the factors that people seek out. Many viewers in India have pigged out on foreign MasterChef shows and one would like to attribute it to the perfection in plated presentation, quite apart from the setting, tempo and quality of culinary preparations that are its raison d'être. Some of the judges, particularly the women, are a picture of perfection even when they are wolfing down mouthfuls. Our regional MasterChef all-male-judges shows also have presenters who are smartly turned out with an attitude to match—combining the eagle-eyed, the empathetic, and the elegant to keep contestants in awe and make net audiences drool.

For the corporate honchos, men and women need to do more than just put their best foot forward. The best face must be assumed for the faces you encounter—to land that order, bag a new client, find a biz partner. If, on the other hand, it is the boss who is in focus, he or she needs to be equally in tune and tone and not take the position for granted. The desire to go from local to global, to have an enhanced executive presence, to become a knowledge-ready leader is what has defined the successful CEO.

To find these qualities of being perspicacious, ever in front-step mode, as world citizens, and to top it all, acing the presentability quotient, is a couple I have chosen to highlight on these pages. They warrant mention here on a number of counts. They are both from the Indian Administrative Service—bureaucrats of a high calibre that gives them the extra edge in the assignments they have chosen to helm.

Dipa Bagai has been an international civil servant with the United Nations and was the Regional Team Leader for Knowledge, Innovation and Capacity Development in UNDP Asia Pacific in Bangkok, and worked with the regional offices of the World Bank in Paris and Bangkok, and with the Government of India on governance and human development programmes.

Atul Bagai, as India Head of the United Nations Environment Programme, works on a multitude of environmental challenges in India, including out-of-the-box initiatives such as a sustainable textile hub for India. He was instrumental in designing and developing synergies between Ozone Depleting Substance phase-out and climate change in 41 countries of Asia and Pacific as the UNEP Senior Regional Coordinator.

They are true ambassadors for India. In their in-depth knowledge of Indian tradition—music, food, textiles, art, literature—the list is legion. I saw them in action during the tenure of their assignment in Southeast Asia, how they conducted themselves with dignity, reached out to the local populace through their classy entertaining style, and supported many projects. With them, substance has married style. Their unique dress sense has made them project the country in the most subtle ways—Atul Bagai in his Lucknowi chikan kurtas that he wears regularly to office, and Dipa Bagai in her mostly off-white, finely woven and hand embroidered sarees—both supporting the Sewa movement in their homeland, Lucknow. However, over the years, Dipa Bagai has developed her own style, wearing a formal handloom sarong with a structured top, when she travels. This ensures that she can step off the plane and into a boardroom and look snappy, sorted and traditional to the hilt.

Making their mark with presentability are all the bankers who are our relationship managers and have their work cut out to keep up a financial interface. What I admire about them is the natty dressing, even in the hottest weather, which shows their commitment and gives me an incentive to give them the time of day. They may often go back empty-handed, but a smart impression is a valuable investment for another day.

While the idea of Friday dressing has been capitalized on by shirt manufacturers, a certain informality was introduced into the regimented workweek, but the question always remained for the female workforce. What were they supposed to wear? In one of the multinationals where I had worked, men were encouraged to come in T-shirts and bush shirts on Saturdays. But where did the handful of women executives fit into these 'rules'? I was always in sarees, so I thought Saturday could mean salwaar-kameez. But no—although this had considerably more coverage than a saree, it did not fit in with what male bosses were accustomed to. One of the Canadian directors commented wryly that if women in sarees showing their midriff could be accepted, the full coverage of the 'Punjabi outfit' was a darned sight more modest. At the end, men continued with their casual wear, the lone exception being a colleague who would always come in a crisp dhoti and kurta. What an elegant statement of regional pride!

In my later avatar as a consultant, I tweaked it so that I could wear western formals—jackets and trousers, particularly in the cooler months, and the acceptability came with some grudging appreciation thrown in. Everything has changed today, though. Indo-Westerns have given a wide berth to women's choices and edges have blurred with dressing that is unisex. Designers have come up with novel approaches and mix and match gives immense flexibility.

However, it is our airlines that have written new sets of dress code for their crew members, and here, I focus on female flight attendants. The swishing silk sarees with high-backed air-hostess *choli*s continue apace for Indian airlines, while on the other hand, there are the new-age airlines which have a set of crew where women are in skirts, trousers, smart blouses and customized hairstyles. An international look and perfect eye candy for the harried traveller and definitely the right attitudinal construct.

Professional couturists, we found, came on board to design uniforms for various airlines. Indigo got Rajesh Pratap Singh, who designed the navy-blue uniforms. They went a step further with the makeup styling done by Ambika Pillai, who even did further detailing on specific lipstick and nail polish shades. There were regulations over short wigs or a bun look, and they sported an air of efficiency in keeping with their on-time philosophy.

But announcements must undergo a huge course correction. Some airlines paper over the problem by getting professional voices to make initial announcements. Yet more effort has to be made to train crew in all languages to speak clearly, enunciate better and pronounce city names with authenticity.

My cavil at the end of the day is also this—dress codes are fabulous brand builders and make for confidence instilled in passengers and clients, but what about hiring experts to teach them interpersonal skills, communicative techniques, thinking on their feet (literally!). Apart from their training on voice, accent, deportment, articulation and maintaining a positive exterior, are they taught to interact with fellow colleagues in a non-aggressive manner, or handle the ever-irate and ready-to-criticize passenger?

Coming to the defence of the importance given to attitude, and not just appearance, was Sanjiv Kapoor, a veteran of the aviation industry, who had played a major role in the turnaround of SpiceJet and later headed Vistara as its chief strategy and commercial officer, seeing it through a major period of growth. In my interaction with him, he was seized of the fact that politeness, courtesy and the importance of empathy and human decency were key elements the airline stressed on, as also in the handling of unruly, unseemly passengers. Safety training, guest instructors, grooming specialists—all of these contribute to the attitude code in his opinion.

There could not be any element of fluke in the actions of cabin crew. They would have to do unto passengers as they themselves would want to be treated. The aircraft had to be looked at as their home; they would have to serve in the best manner, keep it tidy, and have pride in service and upkeep and upscaled conduct.

But going back to dress code, we gathered that Vistara had got Abraham and Thakore to design uniforms for the cabin crew, with the brief that it had to be practical, distinctive and outstanding from a global branding perspective—with a blend of Asian, Indian and Western. The aubergine was an unusual colour, it stood out at airports and the whole outlook was aimed at showing a global Indian citizen—the international Indian.

The crew of Vistara got into the retro act when they were paying tribute to the JRD Tata legacy. Their livery represented the golden age of flying, with the cabin crew wearing uniforms from the '50s and '60s inspired by Jackie O, while an aircraft was painted in the colours of the original Tata Air Lines of the 1930s. It got a lot of traction.

He rewound to the time when SpiceJet was going through a downturn. Kapoor was instrumental in the unimaginable turnaround story. There is one quirky action that got them great mileage, and its share of criticism too. Kapoor recalls how during Holi in 2014, the crew greeted passengers with a *tika* and as the plane took off, they did a peppy 'Balam Pichkari' dance number that got all passengers smiling and a few even joined the crew. Kapoor was quick to add that the crew was additional to the on-duty one, and had been trained to dance so that they moved gracefully and not excessively. When the DGCA issued a show cause notice over compromising safety, the airline answered that they had Boeing do a study which showed that moving a meal cart down the aisle would have had a greater impact than the crew dancing down it. People had taken out their cell phones to record the moment and it was only after that incident and publicity that permissions were finally given for phones to be permitted on-board in airplane mode, repealing an outdated regulation.

Following the celebrated Holi dance, Kapoor got a call from the then promoter, who asked him, 'You made the cabin crew dance?' Expecting a dressing down, Kapoor was surprised when the promoter said: 'Do one thing—make them dance every day, sales have shot through the roof!'

And there is one more aspect—not just how much you expect of your employees, your crew members, but also what you can give in return by way of loyally backing their actions. So, when someone tweeted a picture of an air hostess napping at the Bengaluru airport lounge and tagged Kapoor in the post, he staunchly backed her. When I asked him about the incident, he said, the air hostess was on a break between flights and briefly fell asleep and in any case, the lounge was provided for the crew to rest in. His riposte: 'We do not condone such photos being taken of our crew or customers without their permission, nor do we think it is correct to post such photos on social media. Our crews are the finest in the industry and are human too.'

The picture was taken down without demur immediately. Social media users were all praise for this action and some said that he was the kind of boss they would love to work for.

So, thinking creatively and acting with empathy could gain you satisfaction mileage in the long haul, if executed with thought.

Talking about credibility and the customer acceptance factor, high-end restaurants and hotels of repute are hiring designers to come up with distinctive wear for their service staff. The renowned design duo Lecoanet–Hemant look at factors like the standard and the vision of the hotel and the way the hotel wants to be perceived. 'Some are very classical and traditional; some are much more contemporary and modern.' 'Some want to treat the client as god, some want to treat the client as a friend who is visiting,' is how they minutely approach the creation of uniforms.

But in tandem with the design element, the need is for hotels to get professionals to train frontline staff to speak, to pronounce impossible names of dishes, to become au fait with culinary terms, and of course, manage the daily complaints that are an inevitable fallout in the service industry.

Changing parameters in attitude also determine what people are prepared to accept in the visual medium. Television newscasters, particularly women, have perfected their individual 'looks', whether in the studio or on the field.

Sports presenters, and here I mention the new clutch of women, have got their viewers to accept their long-legged looks and curvatures, giving prop to the notion that knowledge of the game's fine, but you must also add the oomph factor.

Going into such mundane detailing is only to labour a point—the appropriateness of apparel to sync with the occasion and the institutional ambience. One of our governor's wives, in West Bengal, would dress informally when we were invited to dine with them.

But the moment she had to take a plane ride, it was always classic sarees and shawls, in keeping with the high official status. I always admired former West Bengal governor M.K. Narayanan, who proudly wore his mundu at all official functions and was the picture of male elegance.

In summary, **attitude, apparel and altitude are the three sides of an isosceles triangle that make up the credibility quotient**.

23

Webpage: Of Social Media and Societal Connect

If you wish the social media to gainfully ply
Which will make you the successful web-winged gadfly
You can get a quick fix
But it really will nix
All the real-time chinwags that have communion comply

In Bengal, the famous coffee house *adda* is no longer part of our oeuvre. The plaintive song which was sung by the internationally acclaimed playback singer Manna Dey, 'Coffee Houser sei addata aaj aar nei', is hummed by all and sundry, and only makes for regrets at the connectivity chat-ful, argumentative days gone by. Now is the generation that is part of a wired, cloud-computing world where all communing is so fleeting, so transactional. And talking of coffee houses, they are growing apace, in sophistication and sophistry, where you look first for a connection to your laptop, then check on the WiFi signals, and then sit with friends, to chat, but all the while, with phone in hand, just so that important WhatsApp message is not missed.

Look at me! Listen to me! Love me! I am live! This is how easily FB, Twitter, Instagram and all else in the social media space allows individuals to whip up their image. It's easy, fast, inexpensive. Your time starts now.

Is all this really transitory, or is it the need of the hour, the trend of our times? We have to be open to everything that could arm us to be visible, audible and 'followable'. But is this the best way to reach our messages in the corporate world, or communicate at an individual level?

For those of us who have had our dietary basics fed on traditional approaches to media, this leap forward has made us do a running jump into the next level of social media platforms in order to stay relevant, connected, ahead. However, in our discussion in this particular chapter, we will present both viewpoints. Not to see which one—the trad or the trending—is winning, but how we feel they should cohabit.

Cloud conversations are necessarily objects thrown at one another, often sifting through personal glories to slosh them on FB 'friends'. But is this making for a real connectivity, a carved-out space for personalized interactivity? Quite the converse, or reverse, we may say. The various tools of social media could be a quick fix for marketing products, doing self-serving promos, cutting corners for PR and advertising efforts through bypassing the print behemoth. It is the butterfly that is beyond social—it soars fast, but often, like the moth that desires the star, it is like the unreachable goals that Shelley prosodied about.

So what are we advocating? The stolid back to basics of people-to-people chatter, confrontation, and an ideological cabal too.

But in doing so, we are looking at both sides of social and societal. Social media, if used judiciously, could be a powerful tool for brand building. For those who are trying to project the image of companies on behalf of their clients, a sure-fire way to ensure targeted audiences. Is this merely a hit-and-miss set of operations, or is there a strategic methodology behind the use of social media?

Tericom co-founders Ritusmita Biswas and Tehnaz Dastoor state, 'Social media is not only a means of quick recognition but also a necessity in today's world. There is no escape from social media—today, even before a journalist writes a story, he will check out the digital media profile of the client. So, before PR or any other offline media begins, your social media credentials need to be perfect.

'The question is whether a brand even exists if it is not on social media? We have used these networking platforms to plant information about clients and build a brand image that is aligned with its communication strategy. Whatever you say in your offline communication—be it advertising or PR-oriented—must be synced with your online communication.'

Both work in tandem and you can survive by just being an online brand, but you cannot survive just being an offline brand anymore. In fact, the tried-and-tested methods of promotions need to be validated now with an online presence, without which the brand loses credibility. 'As brand strategists, we always recommend brands to start with an online presence before they move to any other means of promotions.'

Do events-based strategies work for true impact?

'The events-based approach is a perfect way to integrate online and offline marketing activities. An event with promotions is the best way to build a brand; however, unless it is covered by the media, it does not have any value. Today, though, all the media houses have their social media handles and online editions which are very active. So, even before it goes on print or any offline communication is done about the event, it goes out on the social media handles of the publications or of the influencers, thus reaching its right target audience.'

They believe, as do many of the agencies who are in this space, that events and sponsorship of these are one way of showcasing a company's CSR involvement, be it in arts and crafts, music, literature, or health, nutrition, education programmes, or promoting vocational and economic activities among the lower social-economic strata. It is through these events which are widely covered by the media that society knows about a company's involvement in helping the less fortunate and what it has done for the upliftment of certain sections of society.

'Social media promotion is the only kind which is sustainable,' feels Biswas, whose agency, Digital Brandz, parallelly weighs in with boosting the presence of brands in digital space. She agrees particularly with the fact that what goes once on digital media, stays there. Memories remain on iCloud. 'But if it is well circulated, it stays on various platforms. In fact, if there is any incorrect information planted on digital media, it is very tough to get rid of it permanently.' They are in full sync with the sustainability of social media as the need of the hour.

But for us traditionalists, we constantly keep harping on the need for more societal interaction, which agencies, like Tericom, with high-level contacts could capitalize on. This is a point on which there is no debate at all.

Biswas adds: 'I believe that for PR or social media work, one needs to have a pleasing and outgoing personality. This is then enhanced through a willingness to go out and meet with people (not so much these days though) and continue to build your contacts. Whether it is in the social clubs or being a member of different societies, these contacts are extremely important in life. Being a member of business bodies or having access to them is also an advantage. Obviously, having the right "background" always helps as you can then leverage this to get larger sponsorships, governmental contracts, and work in general.'

Ah! This smacks of the famous old-boy network which worked wonders in the corporate world of the '60s and '70s. It wasn't so much as what you knew but who you knew—golfing buddies, drinking pals, family connections, fellow students and teachers from prestigious schools. These were the lifeblood for job openings and hierarchy hedging. Nothing's really gone away; it's just that the networking is so virtually netted now.

Our book keeps on harking back to the presentability element—for the agencies and their chosen representatives. There are two aspects—one about the intelligence, deportment, dependability, credibility, combined with the right physical look to be able to connect with new clients they are pitching for, and the other, about how they should prime clients to exhibit their best face.

Dastoor concurs: 'It is extremely important to have the "right" staff when dealing with corporate or higher-end clients. Your own deportment, spoken English and presentability are extremely important in making the right impression. Obviously, you must also do your homework prior to meeting with the client so that you are aware of their aesthetic sensibilities and the kinds of information which they have shared in the public domain. This forms an immediate connect with the client and then you can go on presenting your points of view towards enhancing their products/information, etc. Dressing shabbily and speaking in poor English (or in whichever language you are making your presentation) with no homework done, I believe, show your disrespect towards others. Further, it is important for the client to know of similar campaigns which you have undertaken and their success factor when you are presenting your ideas to them.

'Today, we have induced a number of clients to undertake personal branding in the social media and PR space. This is extremely important especially in family-owned second- and third-generation businesses, where the founder or fathers are known to the public and their children less so. Having different ideas and choosing a varied path from the older generation, the younger members want to establish their own identities both as individuals as well as with regard to the new product lines which they want to introduce to the public.'

Though we believe that nothing can beat social interaction, yet today's person-to-person communication has leaped into Microsoft Teams meetings, Zoom sessions, online meetings, across international borders, all of these dictated by Covid-related restrictions, which, to look at the upside, has actually made for better eye contact and pinpointed agendas. Hundreds and thousands of like-minded groups now share information on WhatsApp, book clubs have traversed time and place, Clubhouse gets people chatting for hours on innumerable topics, Zoom plays have removed stage fright, and films have been put together from multiple locations, in an integrated whole.

But combine offline and online, and you have a winner, often—as it happened with an offline campaign of Austin Plywood which was integrated into an online blitz undertaken by Tericom. This agency provides 360-degree solutions, which involve social media, event planning, PR, branding, content and design, website development, social influencing and blogger collaborations, and a full-scale end-to-end conceptualization of campaign strategies.

So, they used these multiple skills, got South Indian superstar Prakash Raj on board, as Austin has a strong market in Hyderabad, and this offline campaign was converted into a large social media and PR campaign in the east. Austin's online followers increased from 350 to over 1.5 lakh with this multimedia campaign, by using billboards, print adverts, and social media platforms. We were witness to this, and the take-home value of the notebooks with the logo has served as a brand reminder.

But at the end of the day, we have to get digital. One would bow down to a Canva or a Hootsuite or a Buffer to go into professional marketing, or zip through an A to Z of social networking services, from About.me to zoo.gr, to get the right vibes, the loudest fit. In fact, one would say, never underestimate the power of Hootsuite. It is a social media management system for businesses and organizations to collaboratively launch and manage campaigns across multiple social networks from a SaaS dashboard. Features include scheduling, monitoring, content creation, analytics, team management, security, and boosting. It helps brands identify customer issues, resolve problems effectively, and create advocates.

The biggest news for India came when Google pledged ₹75,000 crore for an India Digitization Fund, thus accelerating India's digital economy. Making the announcement, Sundar Pichai, the CEO of Google and parent brand Alphabet, talked about how there was a lot of work to be done in order to make the internet 'affordable and useful for a billion Indians, from improving voice input and computing for all of India's languages, to inspiring and supporting a whole new generation of entrepreneurs.' And Google's country head Sanjay Gupta believed that with more Indians learning to do things digitally, 'there is a need to digitally solve the challenges that India faces in health, education or agriculture. More businesses need to be connected and bring digital to their core offer.'

The areas of digitization that are intended to be covered in the next five to seven years are the enabling of affordable access to information in a number of native languages; building products and services to suit the unique needs of Indian demography; using AI for social good in areas such as health, education, and agriculture; and helping small and mid-size businesses to migrate to greater digitalization.

With Google signing an agreement to invest ₹33.7 crore in Jio Platforms, there is a pact to jointly develop an entry-level affordable smartphone with optimizations to the Android operating system and the Play Store. With millions being able to access such smartphones, there is the larger picture of unlocking new opportunities and 'further power the vibrant ecosystem of applications and push innovation to drive growth for the new Indian economy.'

The friendly roadside dhaba and the harried rickshaw puller now willingly accept payments, not with soiled notes of small denominations, but through the magic of GPay. Here, the societal interaction, the knots of people exchanging chai and chatter still continue, and digital zooms into their lives when needed.

24

Weightage: Reimagining Brand Strategies Post Pandemic

A person, a country, a product, acquires the status of brand
When its USP and marketing can on firm perception stand
There's an art to it all
And a scientific stall
That makes for the credible and complete band at hand

The Biswa Bangla logo is omnipresent. We experience it as we steer through the Biswa Bangla Sarani; we consume its handloom and handicrafts at the Biswa Bangla stores in Kolkata and at the airport; it shouted out its standing prominently at the Global Business Meet, was emblazoned at the Fifa Under-17 Football World Cup, and showed up on awards dispensed by the state. Designed uniquely by the chief minister herself, it is graphically strong and it proclaims proudly: 'Where the World Meets Bengal'. Under the Biswa Bangla umbrella, the best of weaving, art and craft has been sourced and marketed, benefitting millions of artisans.

Puff prelims accounted for, the larger question looms: After attracting so many eyeballs and garnering a lot of goodwill, shouldn't this logo become the basis for a bigger push to envelop it all into a macro-branding for the state's persona? Having had a resounding victory in the elections, the ruling party today could be looking at a new set of strategies to promote and rebrand the state. During the pandemic, with so many other pressing healthcare issues at stake, can, and should, a state take a long-term relook at projecting its capabilities, considering the rerouting of investors to the state, a revival of the core industries, and a revalidation of tourism?

Yet, when it comes to spelling out the innate qualities and values of the state as a brand, we are confused. Are we the cultural core of the country or the state with complete touristic trappings? Are we the gateway to the East, or do we project a heritage halo?

To get a deeper understanding of the issue, we sought out brand guru Harish Bijoor, also known as a strategy consultant and disruption evangelist in the corporate space. During the pandemic, he had advised companies not to shut shop. So, how would he look at the marketing of the state in the long term? Another question that we slid into its slipstream: does a brand ambassador really add value to the image of a state? We are personally wary of the countries or cities or states that 'use' a brand ambassador, cost no concern, to give heft to their own vanities. An exception, possibly, was the Shah Rukh Khan *Be My Guest* Dubai ad, partly because he himself owns a home in the prestigious Palm archipelago, and the incredulous reactions of the populace in the situations where he appeared.

His advice on branding any state at this juncture is to move with caution, and without upsetting the applecart of fearful sentiments that citizens are going through. The planning for brand projection can start, but the execution should await better times.

As for brand ambassadors to promote states, Bijoor feels that they need to be coached into believing in the place that they endorse, heavy advertising notwithstanding. Actors mostly are chosen for their popularity quotient, but the commensurate fee tends to be humungous. He would rather have micro-brand ambassadors, where instead of spending a heap of money on one star, a smaller amount could be spent on more stars and influencers.

Coming to the brands of corporates that he deals with, he has worked out a series of attributes. 'A brand has life and therefore it has a persona. I set out twelve attributes for the brand. Then I try to find people who would endorse. I list out attributes of the endorser. It can be a Shah Rukh Khan or a Sourav Ganguly. I just need to take on people who have a 95 per cent match.'

Bijoor, however, has a greater vision for branding countries. I remember Wally Olins, whom I interacted with during his visits to Kolkata, talking about branding Spain, even getting artist Joan Miro to do a fanciful logo, gratis, being the proud Spaniard that he was.

But here, Bijoor has some very keen observations on nation branding. 'Let's look at Brand India,' he says. 'It is a nation for a start: a robust nation that packs in the energies of a billion, plus a third of a billion, people. Brands have two aspects to concern themselves with. One is an intrinsic one. What do people within the country think of Brand India? The second is an extrinsic one: What do countries outside India think of our nation? And more importantly, from today's context, what do the 6.3 billion people who live in these countries think of India? Do they think differently from what their governments want them to think of India the nation?'

'The current theme "Incredible India" has served the nation long enough now, with its very visual emphasis on everything that is fantastic and nice in India. My research probe tells me that the phrase does well for India Tourism, but not necessarily for Brand India.

'"Incredible India" is a phrase that cuts both ways in positivity and negativity, depending on the experiences of people with the nation. I do believe we need to pave the way for a powerful, reliable, consistent and "Credible India" as opposed to an "Incredible India" as the current theme puts it.

'The world went through the throes of tumult that the pandemic brought into our lives. People in every nation went through uncertainty of every kind. Volatility was the norm, and the minds of people all across grappled to clutch on to the rays of hope that emerged from anywhere and everywhere.

'Countries of every kind went through the phases of fear and panic. Now, as the economy of hope emerges ahead, it just might be the right time for India to reposition itself correctly and strongly in the minds of the world at large. What the world thinks of India, and more importantly, what the people who live in these many countries all across think of India is going to define our nation brand.

'Isn't it time we stopped saying "Made in India" on our products and services that find their way across the world? It is time to do it the "Swiss way". Why not use the "India Made" phrase all across?

'"Made in India" means made in a geography that is India. It doesn't mean much. 'India Made', on the other hand, means made by the proud Indian with hard work, effort, and most importantly, with India-passion poured into it!'

Another aspect troubles us in the context of entrepreneurs—who understand the science and nuts and bolts of starting up their businesses but do not set any store by the art and philosophy of branding. Does this lacuna present an opportunity for brand experts?

There is a broader ecosystem of entrepreneurs. The numbers are huge—maybe around 63 million. Bijoor says: 'We are actually a nation of entrepreneurs. Everyone and their uncle is one. But each one is a competent persona. Most of the business is a physical brick-and-mortar business. The DNA is putting together a business. Unfortunately, there is no proportionate element of communication in it. Entrepreneurs feel that after I produce I am not really concerned about the communication. Competence of production needs the competence of communication. It only comes when they realize that they have to reach out to a consumer by using the right decibel and the right tenor—everything that is part of communication science. Entrepreneurs view it merely as an art, whereas there is a deeper philosophy and scientific approach that goes with the creation of a product or an idea. Communication must be straightforward and it must go to the heart of the consumer. Everyone must get it into their DNA. It must be a part of the first bit of entrepreneurship.

'If you look at the fact that a typical brand strategy person is approached at the last minute, I would call it a crime of omission and commission. It shows that you do not respect the totality of your own business. You have to believe in the totality of your communication. There is no one-size-fits-all strategy or a cut-and-paste branding. The brand partner must go into the DNA of the setup and create a USP.' As a brand expert, he has often refused large clients, even multinationals, who look for a quick fix.

Going on to brand building for individuals, can it stand the test of time? This refers to political figures and people in the entertainment industry. Since our book is all about presentability and the perfection quotient, can this be an important aspect of the total package that is projected of an individual? Could an individual be bigger than the product? It certainly did in the political arena. Jayalalitha, a six-term chief minister in Tamil Nadu, saw her Amma brand of affordable products and services, including water and cement and salt to name just part of the slew of initiatives, resonate with the masses in her state, with her much publicized Amma canteens providing cheap and nourishing fare. She became an iconic, much worshipped, if at times controversial, figure—the iron lady whose face and personality dominated over a considerable length of her tenure. *Thalaivii*, a biographical film made with a reported ₹100-crore budget with actress Kangana Ranaut essaying her role, continues to keep her personal life alive.

In West Bengal, Chief Minister Mamata Banerjee's personality as 'Didi' has had the same brand impact, with some large-scale initiatives to benefit women and children and the rural populace, and her hoardings and cut-outs projecting the benevolent face of the CM. Didi's reach-out schemes for women have gained her much support. Here, too, the dominance of the people's CM, in her simple cotton sarees and chappals, but with a strong voice, is possibly the brand in which the general public find a credible support for their needs and aspirations.

Another powerful brand—again a woman—an individual larger than her designation as chief minister of one of our most populous states, Uttar Pradesh, has been Mayawati, who has served four separate terms and who is affectionately referred to as Behenji, a sister. Her welfare schemes, like the other chief ministers mentioned here, were aimed at the poor and downtrodden people of the state, in the process spending several thousand crores. Her birthdays were massively media-connect events, where she would appear dripping in diamonds. The *Time* magazine included her in India's most influential list. However, her creation of larger-than-life-size statues of Buddhist and Hindu, Dalit and OBC figures, herself included in this list, attracted a lot of attention, but also swathes of criticism.

If we move on to other 'influential' individuals, this time in the corporate sector, the one name that stands out is Vijay Mallya, the 'King of Good Times'. Bijoor opines, 'His persona was built to show him greater than he was. His personal branding was so heavy that it overshadowed everything around him.' But there must be a sense of integrity. 'Politicians and sports stars are told that they would not be represented in the wrong manner. If you are a wolf, brand yourself as a wolf and not a wolf in sheep's clothing. Brand yourself as someone with anger issues, for instance. That is your uniqueness.'

His entire approach to the branding of any celebrity, like a cricketer, has been to live with him for a couple of days and be a fly on the wall. Two days is enough to understand the real person, the core of his personality. He gives the analogy of how a dosa in every home has holes in it, but each house will have a different look and consistency. Thus, that is how he has managed to extract confessions and find latent faults, and in totality, make a credible brand emerge.

Having gone through such exercises, how are clients convinced about their return on investment? There are two kinds of clients—one kind who expect immediate returns. They have the transactional trader mindset. 'Unfortunately, you cannot expect this when it comes to people. A brand is a thought that lives in a person's mind. A thought is not a solid item. A thought is the mind of a consumer. Thoughts come and change and die and at the same time, the environment in which a thought lives is the mind. I like to give the example of cricketer Virat Kohli who to me is a brand. He is a thought which lives in people's minds. But in every person's mind, it is different. That is what I term as the complexity of branding. You need to plant the thought in a person's mind. You devein it of the extra thoughts. You plant a seed and wait for it to mature. It is a tree that takes time to grow. If you look at the four Ps of marketing strategy, the fifth P would be patience. You commit yourself to a brand in the long term.'

Going on to the next level of communication, and in the new normal of locked-down challenges, it would appear that digital is here to stay.

Bijoor philosophises: 'Home-centric makes you digital. Whether it is real estate, print and travel and other industries—digital lives in pure existence in our lives. Digital gives you something free and takes back more. Digital will coagulate and command eventually. The consumer's propensity to go digital has received a nudge as never before. There is no going back from the domino effect of this nudge.'

Most of us have a deep-seated optimism about the post-pandemic scenario. Meanwhile, digital, virtual or any other form of communication will keep our hopes up and businesses at the ready. 2022 and beyond—2025 to be precise, when this book sees the light of day—promises fresh outlooks.